Female Genital Cosmetic Surgery

Female Genital Cosmetic Surgery

Solution to What Problem?

Edited by

Sarah M. Creighton
University College London Hospitals

Lih-Mei Liao
University College London Hospitals

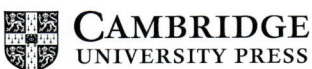
CAMBRIDGE
UNIVERSITY PRESS

CAMBRIDGE
UNIVERSITY PRESS

University Printing House, Cambridge CB2 8BS, United Kingdom

One Liberty Plaza, 20th Floor, New York, NY 10006, USA

477 Williamstown Road, Port Melbourne, VIC 3207, Australia

314–321, 3rd Floor, Plot 3, Splendor Forum, Jasola District Centre, New Delhi – 110025, India

79 Anson Road, #06–04/06, Singapore 079906

Cambridge University Press is part of the University of Cambridge.

It furthers the University's mission by disseminating knowledge in the pursuit of
education, learning, and research at the highest international levels of excellence.

www.cambridge.org
Information on this title: www.cambridge.org/9781108435529
DOI: 10.1017/9781108394673

© Sarah Creighton and Lih-Mei Liao 2019

First published 2019

Printed and bound in Great Britain by Clays Ltd, Elcograf S.p.A.

A catalogue record for this publication is available from the British Library.

Library of Congress Cataloging-in-Publication Data
Names: Creighton, Sarah M., editor. | Liao, Lih-Mei, editor.
Title: Female genital cosmetic surgery : solution to what problem? / edited by Sarah M. Creighton, Lih-Mei Liao.
Description: Cambridge, United Kingdom ; New York, NY : Cambridge University Press, 2018. | Includes bibliographical
references and index.
Identifiers: LCCN 2018046098 | ISBN 9781108435529 (pbk. : alk. paper)
Subjects: | MESH: Gynecologic Surgical Procedures | Reconstructive Surgical Procedures – methods | Reconstructive
Surgical Procedures – ethics | Genitalia, Female – surgery | Body Image
Classification: LCC RD119 | NLM WP 660 | DDC 617.9/52–dc23
LC record available at https://lccn.loc.gov/2018046098

ISBN 978-1-108-43552-9 Paperback

....

Contents

Contributors

Jennifer Beale, MBBS, FRANZCOG
King Edward Memorial Hospital and
Perth Children's Hospital
Perth, Australia

Virginia Braun, PhD
University of Auckland
Auckland, Āotearoa, New Zealand

Lori A. Brotto, PhD
University of British Columbia
Vancouver, Canada

Maggie Bryce, BA
University of British Columbia
Vancouver, Canada

Clare Chambers, DPhil
University of Cambridge
Cambridge, UK

Hera Cook, PhD
University of Otago Wellington Medical School
Wellington, New Zealand

Sarah M. Creighton, MD, FRCOG
University College London Hospitals
London, UK

Naomi S. Crouch, MD, MRCOG
St Michael's Hospital
Bristol, UK

Brian D. Earp, MSc, MPhil
Yale University and The Hastings Centre
New Haven, CT, USA

Angelica Kavouni Ion, MD, PhD, FRCS(Eng), EBOPRAS
Phoenix Hospital Group
London, UK

Lih-Mei Liao, PhD, FBPsS
University College London Hospitals
London, UK

Tove Lundberg, PhD
Lund University
Lund, Sweden

Lina Michala, PhD, MRCOG
National and Kapodistrian University
of Athens
Athens, Greece

Yana Richens, OBE, PhD, RM
University College London Hospitals
London, UK

Sarah B. Rodriguez, PhD
Northwestern University
Evanston, IL, USA

Arianne Shahvisi, PhD
Brighton and Sussex Medical School
Brighton, UK

Magdalena Simonis, MBBS, FRACGP, DRANZCOG
University of Melbourne
Carlton, Australia

Leonore Tiefer, PhD
Independent Scholar
New York, NY, USA

Nicole Todd, MD
University of British Columbia
Vancouver, Canada

Louise Williams, Bsc, RN (Child)
University College London Hospitals
London, UK

Chapter

1

Female Genital Cosmetic Surgery
Solution in Pursuit of Problem

Lih-Mei Liao and Sarah M. Creighton

Background

Socially motivated female genital cutting has a long history in Europe. According to social historians, in ancient Rome, metal rings were passed through the labia minora of female slaves to prevent procreation. In medieval England, women in certain social strata were made to wear chastity belts to prevent them from engaging in sexual activities during their husbands' long absences. In Tsarist Russia and nineteenth-century England, France and the United States, clitoridectomy was performed to cure epilepsy, hysteria, insanity and masturbation [1]. In many countries today, a diverse range of lawful procedures subsumed under 'female genital cosmetic surgery' (FGCS) overlap with a diverse range of unlawful procedures subsumed under 'female genital mutilation' (FGM) (Chapter 7). The double standard is bewildering:

> How can it be that extensive genital modifications, including reduction of labial and clitoral tissue, are considered acceptable and perfectly legal in many European countries, while those same societies have legislation making female genital cutting illegal, and the World Health Organization bans even the 'pricking' of the female genitals? [2]

FGCS refers to lawful procedures to alter the structure and appearance of female external and internal genitalia in the absence of biomedical concerns. This definition refers to a large and growing number of operations including labiaplasty, clitoroplasty, introitoplasty, hymenoplasty and vaginal rejuvenation, tightening and reconstruction (Chapters 5 and 6). These operations are said to ameliorate women's worries about the appearance and function of their genitals, including the kinds of concerns expressed by our three informants - 'Madison', 'Kate' and 'Navaeh':

> Madison is sobbing. Next to her is her mother Nicole. Opposite them is the gynaecologist who has just examined Madison's vulva. The twenty-year-old has been complaining about soreness from the chaffing and rubbing of her vulva, especially when she wears her jeans. "It gets caught coz it sticks out too much," she says. She has recently cancelled a beach holiday with friends because, she says, her clitoris gets erect in hot weather and can be seen inside her swimwear. Far from feeling relieved by the gynaecologist's reassurance that her genitals are normal and healthy, Madison is miserable. Mother and daughter have spent months researching on the internet before concluding that surgical removal of "the excess tissue" (in the clitoris) was the right course of action for Madison. To Nicole, the persistent despair of her daughter is surely evidence enough that the problem is "not just in her head". Having had a private neck lift herself a few years ago, Nicole is aware of the high costs of private cosmetic surgery and bemoans the fact that it would take Madison years of working at the hair salon to save up enough money to "make the vagina right again".

> Kate lives alone. Her son and daughters live with their respective partners not far away. Kate's husband moved out last year; their divorce has just come through. After several years of stress over the uncertainty of her "rocky marriage", Kate is enjoying life again. She feels ready for a new relationship. After a routine smear test, she asks the friendly nurse about 'vaginal laxity'. It has been at the back of Kate's mind for a while to do something about it. For a few years before the divorce, her husband was initiating sex less often. When they had intercourse, he did not always orgasm. Kate took this to mean that sex with her was less enjoyable for him. Having given birth three times and being post-menopausal, she muses, her body "is bound to feel not as nice". In preparation for a new relationship, and as an act of doing something positive for herself, Kate is looking to see a doctor experienced in 'vaginal tightening'. She wants to know more about the procedure so as to be able to choose the best provider.

> After a successful term at school where she is a high achiever, Nevaeh is excited about her summer travels.

She buys her first pot of hot wax. At fourteen years of age, she is not the first among her friends to remove the unwanted hair growth on her legs. Nevaeh tries on her new bikini and notices her pubic hair escaping through the sides of her briefs. She instinctively proceeds to trim the hair off. An hour later, she is waxing her labia majora. It's extremely painful and her vulva is looking rather red. The enlarged hair follicles give the labial skin a pimpled appearance. Images of chicken skin come to mind and bring a sense of disgust. She despises her "purply fleshy" inner labia even more. She experiences a longing for a firm, smooth-skinned and evenly coloured vulva "without all the bits". Nevaeh shuts her eyes and imagines that different vulva and feels a sense of relief. She can't remember where she may have seen such a "vagina" – perhaps as a drawing in a biology book? Nevaeh feels that she would be so happy if she did not have to deal with the body part that is "so not me".

In 2007, we drew attention to the fivefold increase in the number of labiaplasty operations performed in the United Kingdom's National Health Service (NHS) in the preceding decade [3]. The article was not the first commentary on the topic in a medical journal [4], and there had been important feminist scholarship on the subject [5]. Since then, the FGCS industry has expanded considerably. According to a 2016 report by the International Society of Aesthetic Plastic Surgery (ISAPS), 138,033 labiaplasty operations were performed in the preceding year [6]. These figures come from voluntary data submissions and are almost certainly to be underestimates. The overall increase in the number of cosmetic operations in the year was 9%, but the increase for labiaplasty, which had enjoyed the steepest rise, was 45%. The successful mainstreaming of FGCS in high-income countries is mirrored in low- and middle-income countries, as evidenced, for example, by the specialist sessions on Cosmetic Gynaecology and Vaginal Rejuvenation at the All India Congress of Obstetrics and Gynaecology in 2017 and 2018 [7]. We know that there has not been a labial growth spurt worldwide. In any case, research shows that there is no difference in labial dimensions between women seeking and those not seeking labiaplasty [8]. We also know that surgical techniques do not change that quickly. Hence some other factors must account for the growth of labiaplasty. Psychologist and sexologist Leonore Tiefer explained in 2008 that the infinite possibility of disease mongering in consumerist medicine fits comfortably with our free market and encourages the growth of FGCS [9].

Does the sharp rise in labiaplasty [6] reflect successes of marketing campaigns? Have prices fallen as a result of greater competition so that more women can pay for the operation? Are banks encouraging women to take out personal loans for cosmetic surgery? Is there a new social acceptance of female genital cutting in the West and, if so, what are the implications for women and for society? Has female genital dissatisfaction and distress increased? Are these factors linked, and if so, how?

Female Genital Cosmetic Surgery: Solution to What Problem? is an interdisciplinary response to some of the questions asked. The volume combines historical and philosophical analyses and legal, pedagogic and clinical perspectives. Its aim is first to enable researchers to formulate questions about FGCS more strategically. An equally important aim is to enable education and health professionals to develop non-surgical alternatives to address genital dissatisfaction and the resulting distress (Chapters 11 to 15). The book was seeded by the experiences of women and girls who, like Madison, Kate and Nevaeh, experience doubt, concerns, worries, distress and disgust about the appearance and function of their genitals. It is hoped that some of the chapters will be of interest to the women and girls so affected. Although the volume is about FGCS, many of the discussions are relevant to cosmetic surgery more generally, so that some of the chapters may be of interest to wider audiences.

The contributions to the book by leading academic and clinical experts on the topic of FGCS combine to emphasise the critical importance of reframing the most frequently asked question about FGCS: "Why do women do it?" The question pre-locates the answers in the women and encourages the recycling of individualising discourses of free choice, self-improvement and female madness that exonerate FGCS (Chapter 8). These popularised discourses mask the powerful structural underpinnings of a cultural practice that is being promoted more or less unopposed.

In *Power, Interest and Psychology,* clinical psychologist David Smail proposed that to understand unhappiness, we should, rather than gain insight into ourselves, instead cultivate 'outsight' into the world around us, in particular in how social and economic factors mould our thoughts and feelings and organise our choices in ways that are often not obvious [10]. Outsight into FGCS is the aim of this chapter, in which we highlight and problematise the interrelated systemic processes, including (1) binary notions of sex and gender, (2) the pressure of suspect norms, (3) the effects of medical framing, (4) the ambivalent professional responses, and (5) the barriers to establishing high-quality evidence to guide consumer choice and professional practice. We return to our three informants as the discussion progresses and offer suggestions at the end of the chapter on limiting damage.

Binary Genitals

Like other sex characteristics, the genitalia are culturally constructed as discrete and non-overlapping biological entities that confer femaleness and maleness, two forms of existence also constructed as discrete and non-overlapping. The concept of binary sex is not supported by science. Human embryos have the same reproductive and genital structures to start with. Sex differentiation typically begins at about eight weeks of gestation, and a sex-undifferentiated fetus gradually assumes the anatomical structures and appearance of what we think of as female or male. In other words, the tissues that develop into ovaries, womb, vagina, clitoris and labia are the same as those that develop into testes, penis and scrotum. The developmental processes often, but not always, result in a female- or male-typical combination of chromosomes, physiology and anatomy. Nature prefers diversity and delivers a spectrum of possibilities that makes binary sex a myth so hard to sustain that in modern times, surgical interventions have been developed to 'correct' the less differentiated genitals in many Western(ised) societies. Although the genital differences are medically benign, children may undergo a series of genital operations to satisfy adult expectations of normative genital appearance and function. These interventions are increasingly positioned as a violation of human rights [11].

Binary understandings also extend to non-genital sex characteristics. Body hair, for example, is a biological reality of all human beings, but 'hirsutism', defined as 'an excess of body hair in the male distribution' [12], is a medical term applied only to women. Even if we were to accept that hirsutism is a medical condition for women, the distinction between normal and abnormal female hair growth is far from clear-cut. Women's customary hair removal makes it hard to determine the actual distribution of facial and body hair in the general population. Anthropological studies of cultures in which hair removal is unavailable or not practised indicate that women have the potential to develop hair growth in the same regions of the face and the body as men. The difference between men and women in the amount of hair growth has never been quantified. Nevertheless, clinicians have described women's extreme reactions such as shame and 'morbid preoccupation' even with insignificant hair growth. [13]. Nevaeh takes for granted as a *truth* that females have no body hair. It is a social norm that she has internalised and does not question. As she applies hot wax to remove her leg, armpit and pubic hair, she is merely acting on a commonsense understanding – a matter of *fact*, in her cultural context.

Likewise, although many women in the general population have relatively little breast tissue and many men have more, 'gynaecomastia' is a medical term applied only to men. NHS Choices explains that gynaecomastia is a *medical condition* in which boys' and men's breasts swell to become larger than *normal* [14]. The definition of normal is left to the imagination of providers of 'male breast sculpting', which usually involves a combination of liposuction and removal of glanular tissue. Widely advertised in the private sector, surgery supposedly helps men to "look good in a fitted shirt when the meeting gets heated" [15]. Surgery is intended not just to promote confidence in the board room; it is also said to enable men to "look forward to holidays in the sunshine again". [15]. The American Society of Plastic Surgeons (ASPS) reported a 30% increase between 2010 and 2016 in the number of male breast reductions performed [16].

As discussed above, genitals are socially constructed as mutually exclusively female or male. According to a medical report, a large penis in males "has always symbolized strength, virility, power, and domination in relationships." [17]. The claim is not only sexist but, in erasing cultural differences, racist. The claim is also flawed in *always*. The amount of genital mass proportionate to the overall body mass of the idealised male body form in today's pornographic images is different from that in many classical European artistic depictions. In our contemporary world, surgery on the genitals of men includes penile lengthening, penile girth *enhancement*, dual *augmentation* (length and girth enhancement combined), penile glanular enhancement, scrotal web resection and reconstruction. According to plastic surgeons, many men want to know how phalloplasty can improve their self-confidence, sexual relationships and female partners' sexual satisfaction. Despite these alluring suggestions, phalloplasty fell by 28% between 2015 and 2016 and was the least popular form of cosmetic surgery that year (8,434 operations) [6].

Just as male genitalia are constructed as present, external and pendulous, female genitals are constructed as absent and recessed. In other words, women *lack* genitals [18]; they have an internal receptacle instead. Some years ago, at a planning meeting for an academic event on FGCS, the organisers, who were familiar with the debates, requested that we substitute another word for genitals in the title because it was "a horrible word". They asked that we refer to "vagina" instead. The sensibility did not reflect ignorance on the part of the conference organisers, rather a culturally shared sense of incompatibility between *women* and *genitals*. Madison and Nevaeh refer to 'vagina' when they are talking about the clitoris and labia, which are part of the vulva (Chapter 2). In 1995, artist Joani Blank had the foresight to create *Femalia*, a book of photographs of the vulva. Blank wanted to counter the "unfortunate habit that most people have of calling a woman's vulva her vagina". She reasoned, "by teaching our little girls to call their genitals vaginas, we practice a sort of psychic genital mutilation". Blank forewarned that language could be "as powerful and swift as the surgeon's knife". In her words: "What is not named, does not exist."

Binary notions of genitals explain why men, who on average have a greater share of the burden of genital mass, tend not to complain about the kind of rubbing and chaffing of the genitals that bother women, nor are men known to have their genital mass surgically reduced to accommodate sporting activities such as cycling and horseback riding.

Suspect Norms

Historian Hera Cook (Chapter 9) explains that norms emerge in response to cultural beliefs about a given, regularly occurring action or state, and that individuals who do not conform are sanctioned. Social norms are not experienced as norms but taken for granted as reality and common sense and are not questioned. Individuals consciously or non-consciously scrutinise themselves (and others) and steer towards alignment with the taken-for-granted reality. Norms are therefore an effective form of social regulation, and not always in negative ways. The kind of social norms being interrogated here are the appearance norms that contribute to genital

shame and that which are steering some women and girls towards FGCS.

In a classical series of social psychology experiments, researchers demonstrated how appearance norms operate in social contexts [19]. The research participants were randomly assigned to one of three conditions. They were asked to imagine having an allergy, epilepsy or a physical scar. They then interacted with a conversational partner who they believed to be aware of the condition but was in fact unaware of any of the three experimental conditions. The researchers demonstrated that people who believed that they had a visible defect were more sensitive about the conversational partner's behaviour and were more likely to interpret behaviours such as staring as reactions to the assumed physical defect. They also expressed less favourable impressions of the conversational partner thought to be having the reactions.

Few people can escape the pressure of appearance norms, but surveys consistently show that the majority of women are dissatisfied with or distressed by aspects of their physical appearance, so much so that body dissatisfaction and distress are synonymous with being female [20]. Furthermore, the majority of cosmetic operations are performed on women [6].

In the foregoing example, Madison's sense of threat comes from three *facts*: (1) women have flat vulvas; (2) her vulva is not flat enough; and (3) she will be shamed and humiliated if found out. Madison avoids exposure by withdrawing from certain activities until her sense of threat is removed. If she goes ahead with the beach holiday as planned, Madison is, according to the aforementioned psychological research, likely to feel self-conscious and interpret people's behaviours as intrusive. She is likely to think that her genitals have given rise to the unwelcome attention. She may disengage from social interaction. Convinced by her interpretation of the situation, she is not reassured by her friends' alternative explanations. Madison may decide to wear a sarong to the beach to cover up her presumed defect. In this case, her self-judgement is untested. Either way, her norm-based beliefs are maintained.

Gradual changes to sexual experiences and preferences in response to ageing and other life circumstances are not diseases, unless people choose to view them as such. In Kate's (sub)culture, a reduced capacity for orgasm in men contradicts the social norm of undiminished lustful urges in men. To Kate, her observation of the changes in her then husband needs explaining. As an older woman, 'vaginal laxity', not a recognisable condition, medical or otherwise, is culturally available as an explanation. Kate may be sexually experienced enough to know that enjoyable sex does not require a perfect body. She may remember the days when she and her then husband enjoyed coitus not long after she had given birth, so that 'vaginal laxity' is not a logical explanation. Kate may also remember that their relationship was not going well and that this was affecting their overall pattern of physical affection, not just their sexual experiences. Nevertheless, 'vaginal tightening' somehow sounds like a credible solution for something, albeit Kate has not quite thought through what kind of difference the intervention would make to her life and how. Kate may go ahead and benefit from the intervention. Alternatively, she may notice no difference after a while and regret wasting the money. It is also possible that Kate is harmed by the procedure to the extent that she never enjoys vaginal sex again. No one may hear of such an outcome, perhaps not even Kate's surgeon, because she may blame herself and just want to forget the entire episode. In the absence of independent research, no one can be sure what happens to the many women who undergo invasive interventions on their genitals.

It would be inaccurate to claim that the denigration of female genitals is caused by FGCS. In their 2001 research report, psychologists Virginia Braun and Sue Wilkinson identified seven persistent negative representations of the vagina [21]. The authors discussed how these representations had become culturally available resources for how the vagina and its functions were thought of, talked about and acted on. As the denigrating ideas become everyday understandings, they are no longer questioned and shut down other ways of thinking and talking about the vagina. Cultural devaluing of ordinary female genitals contributes to the fertile ground for FGCS to flourish.

Medical Framing

Citing advertisements of beauty products in popular magazines that target women, philosopher Luna Dolezal drew attention to the routine use of medical and scientific jargon in marketing [22]. Moisturising creams are said to be 'clinically tested' to be able to 'fight free radicals', having been developed through 'years of groundbreaking DNA research'. Scientific vocabularies are deployed to validate other types of products too. Certain toothpastes are claimed to be preferred by dentists. Food supplements are often said to contain nutrients more 'bioavailable' than those found in food. Advertisements for cleaning compounds may claim a capability for infection control in ordinary households. Product developers understand the cultural currency enjoyed by medicine and science and how to appropriate the vocabulary.

Medical framing of certain bodily attributes as normal and others as abnormal can have powerful effects on how people think and feel about (their) bodies. Words such as hirsutism and gynaecomastia trump the reality of diverse combinations of female-typical and male-typical sex characteristics in human beings and put pressure on people for self-surveillance, self-judgement and self-regulation of appearance and comportment to fit with cultural norms. The naming of bigger labia as 'labial hypertrophy' or 'luscious lips' constructs two realities that shape different actions and reactions. Even so, not all women who seek FGCS are duped into believing that they have a genital defect such as labial hypertrophy. On the contrary, many women know that they have ordinary genitals that are not especially flawed. Some even say explicitly that their desire to have the interventions is shaped by normative pressures. However, such awareness is not always enough to defend against the unrelenting feelings of being not good enough.

Invasive and irrevocable genital surgery can be justified only if the genitals are considered out of range and medical interventions as normalising (Chapters 7 to 9). Normal has to be redefined if more out of range vulvas were to be created to grow the FGCS industry. Historian Sarah Rodriguez (Chapter 4) accounts for how larger labia have become rarer through the changing conversations in medicine. Women used to be sold the dream vulva that was aspired to but known to be a statistical rarity. Today, they are being sold 'the new normal' (Chapter 3). Rhetorical sculpting both precedes and follows surgical sculpting of female genitalia.

The power of framing on medical decision-making was demonstrated experimentally by a group of researchers in Zurich [23]. These researchers were interested in how parents decide to allow cosmetic genital surgery on their children with medically benign genital differences. The researchers asked medical students to imagine that they were parents of a child born with 'ambiguous genitalia' – genitals not obviously female- or male-typical and with elements of both. Participants were randomly assigned to one of two scenarios which involved watching a video presenting either medicalised information about ambiguous genitalia by an actor claiming to be a physician or de-medicalised information by the same actor claiming to be a psychologist. Participants were then asked whether or not they would consent to corrective surgery for their imagined child. Research participants in the first scenario were three times more likely as those in the second one to choose surgery for their imagined child. Both groups believed that they had decided independently of any undue influence.

Medical framing sanctions norm-induced genital insecurities and simultaneously claims to resolve them. These transactions operate freely in neoliberal consumerist societies that vilify FGM as violence against girls and women. The rhetorical manoeuvre to separate FGCS from FGM by positioning the former as a cure for psychological distress (and therefore a clinical rather than cultural practice) is flimsy and losing credibility increasingly (Chapter 7). As Clare Chambers aptly observes, although supposedly it is legal to operate on healthy genitals only if proven *necessary* for the person's *mental health*, FGCS providers typically do not refer to mental health in their advertisements or state that they operate only on patients mentally troubled by their genitals (Chapter 8).

Professional Ambivalence

In the United Kingdom in 2012, the silicone breast implant scandal exposed woeful lapses in product quality, aftercare and record keeping [24]. About 300,000 women in 65 countries were believed to have received implants made by a French company, the Poly Implant Prothèse (PIP). The PIP implants were filled with industrial grade silicone rather than medical grade material suitable for use in a human body. The implants were twice as likely to burst and had been associated with toxicity. About 47,000 British women were thought to have had PIP implants. Attention was also drawn to the potential costs incurred by the NHS in dealing with the health problems caused by the implants inserted into women mostly by private practitioners.

Professor Sir Bruce Keogh was asked to chair a committee to review the regulation of cosmetic interventions in the United Kingdom. The report was published in 2013 and drew attention to widespread misleading advertising, inappropriate marketing and unsafe practices [25]. The report was especially critical of the lack of regulation with regards to non-surgical cosmetic interventions, stating that "a person having a non-surgical cosmetic intervention has no more protection and redress than someone buying a ballpoint pen or a toothbrush." The purchasing of FGCS and other cosmetic operations hopefully comes with some protection, although the actual amount of accessible protection is hard to quantify. While UK surgical providers have to be registered with the Care Quality Commission, the lack of clear standards for the provision of cosmetic surgery services means that regulatory bodies are unable to perform effective reviews.

With reference to FGCS, the Keogh Report acknowledged the increased demand in recent years and emphasised the need for providers to have a clear understanding of the legislation on FGM, as well as the importance of managing patient expectations. Like other reports, it alluded to the importance of psychological assessment. The idea of psychological assessment and 'education and counselling' [26] is an interesting one. Although body distress and a decision to have cosmetic surgery are psychological processes, the individual seeking surgery can be said to be accessing *psychology with a scalpel*. This makes actual psychological interventions, the kind provided by people with real psychological expertise, rather redundant. Madison may admit to intense preoccupations that are familiar to psychological practitioners, but she may also insist that the strong emotions will disappear with surgery.

The value of nuanced psychological interventions could be explored (Chapters 12 to 14). However, psychological experts may have to negotiate how their input is positioned, to ensure that they can bring tangible psychological benefits for the women and are not mobilised to salvage respectability for consumerist medicine or, worse still, be an alibi for maverick medicine. When surgery is clearly on offer and there is no decision to be made, psychological input is no more than a rubberstamping exercise for FGCS. This would be unproductive and undermining for both psychologist and client.

A number of opinions from professional bodies express reservations about FGCS, but none of them can claim to have had a significant impact on practice. It is understandably challenging for professional bodies to manage the conflicted interests of their memberships. A few years ago, the Royal College of Obstetricians and Gynaecologists (RCOG) established a new ethics committee under the impeccable stewardship of Dame Suzi

Leather. It was our privilege to work alongside leading academics and practitioners and highly experienced lay representatives, to serve a distinguished institution and the general public. The committee's first task was to develop an ethical opinion paper on FGCS, a process that took two years from inception to eventual publication in 2013 [27]. The document had to accommodate multiple revisions. According to the eventual published opinion, labiaplasty performed for 'medical or functional reasons' is ethically unproblematic (despite an absence of medical indications), as opposed to the same operations carried out for 'aesthetic reasons'. Despite the dedicated input of a highly able multidisciplinary committee, the opinion has had no discernable impact. UK providers blatantly advertise for 'aesthetic' FGCS and make no mention of medical indications.

The challenge of managing conflicted interests is unlikely to be unique to any one institution. The influence of partisan interests may well have worked their way into all professional documents on FGCS. Professional opinions are not legally binding. A confident and unambiguous message can guide meaningful reflections and encourage practice improvements without prohibiting FGCS. At the same time that the RCOG paper was launched, the British Society for Paediatric and Adolescent Gynaecology (BritSPAG) released a position statement that expressed a much clearer collective view against performing labiaplasty on girls younger than the age of 18 years [28]. It is a duty of public bodies to centralise the interests of women and girls in the context of contentious practices such as FGCS.

In the United Kingdom, as in many other countries, cosmetic surgery is not a medical specialty in its own right. There is no recognised training and accreditation pathway, a fact that may not be known to many consumers, who may believe that their surgeons have undergone extensive training and supervised practice before being allowed to operate on them. The Keogh Report recommended the introduction of proper standards for training and accreditation. The principles and implementation of bioethics should be threaded through any training programme and continuing professional development. Demonstration of diligence in the application of bioethics principles should be a requirement for renewal of registration. Because cosmetic surgery is justified on the grounds of ill-defined psychological

distress rather than recognisable diseases, a good working knowledge of relevant psychosocial research and methods should also be a learning outcome.

Barriers to Research

Research that yields replicable and generalisable findings to help women make an informed choice is as badly needed as it is unlikely to happen. In the United Kingdom, cosmetic surgery in the private sector was worth £720 million in 2005. Ten years later, the industry was worth an estimated £3.6 billion [25]. At this level of financial reward, it is difficult to imagine how practitioners could afford to spend time in collaborating on complex research studies. However, there are other obstacles.

Post-FGCS, the consumer's subjective appraisal falls along a spectrum of satisfaction and dissatisfaction. For the satisfied customer, the modified genitalia are no longer 'not me'. The idea is not for her to experience her genitalia as artificially constructed but as an assimilated and naturalised part of her. She is not likely to want to participate in longer-term research and be repeatedly reminded of the surgery. The women who are dissatisfied or not wholly satisfied are unlikely to re-engage with their surgeons for additional reasons. Many research reports do not specify attrition rates and those that do suggest that many patients are lost to follow-up (Chapter 6). These shortcomings vastly limit the generalisability of any conclusion. Dissatisfied women are the people whom FGCS providers have the most to learn from. Their scarcity in research deprives practitioners of the opportunities to hear about the limitations of what they do, so that they can adjust their claims and manage their own and their clients' expectations more effectively.

FGCS represents a loose assemblage of controversial procedures that are continually being added to and rebranded to attract new customers, so that any negative research findings can be said to be out of date. That is, providers can argue that techniques have changed and that the problems identified are no longer relevant. These conditions justify the classification of some FGCS procedures as experimental. The design of future research and data handling should therefore involve researchers who operate independently of the service providers and proprietors. If techniques keep changing and the evidence cannot catch up, it is imperative for women and girls like Madison, Kate and Nevaeh to know about the experimental nature of the procedures and make an informed choice.

Limiting Damage

The rise in the number of websites offering FGCS is being shadowed by a rise in the number of websites advertising repeat operations to overcome the problems of *botched labiaplasty* [29], referred to by some providers as "avoidable unintentional female genital mutilation" [30]. The same providers who offer repeat operations also provide primary labiaplasty [29]. All of the services imply that it is providers other than themselves who *botch* women's labia, exhibiting a pattern of self-serving ignorance. A review of the content of the advertisements has identified a lamentable lack of quality information on safety and effectiveness. The same women whose expectations are not met by their primary surgery are now being targeted for more of the same, with no more assurance than verbal claims. For women who undergo repeat genital operations, it is debatable how much more protection and redress they can readily access, compared to those available when buying a ballpoint pen or a toothbrush.

There is no question that FGCS providers need to be made much more accountable. The question is how. High-quality research may never be possible in the field, and the need for research should no longer be deployed to stall the implementation of much more rigorous regulatory measures. Therefore, submission of clinical data to a system designed by an independent, multidisciplinary research group should become mandatory. The findings should be freely accessible to the public. These activities should be funded by the profit-making services.

As well as training in bioethics for providers, a much tighter decision-making protocol for patients should be formulated nationally, to ensure consistency in implementation. Informed consent is an ethical imperative that transcends legal requirements. The principles are outlined by the General Medical Council, which recommends a two-stage process [31]. The period of reflection between stages gives patients the opportunity to consider the full implications of surgery. There can, however, be a gulf between ethical principles and ethical behaviours in this service context

and perhaps cosmetic surgery more generally [32]. The decision to undergo FGCS is to a greater or less extent driven by emotions. The more emotive the situation, the more likely are consumers to selectively attend to the desired outcome and minimise the risks or filter out the potential for disappointment. The chance of a mismatch in understanding between provider and recipient is high. A rigorous protocol should elaborate on risk information and include a discussion of potential problems that have not been properly investigated. If during the consultation the patient is presented with the perfect 'after' images, she should also be shown the imperfect ones. The provider should offer a genuine space for women to discuss no surgery as a valid option, at least for the time being. The woman should be able to repeat back to the provider the risks, benefits and limitations discussed, to ensure that the information is processed. Further questions should of course always be encouraged. However, many women may not know what questions to ask, so that the onus is on the provider to ensure that all the bases are covered [32].

The FGCS industry exists at women's expense, physically, emotionally and financially. By definition it can grow only with more women feeling worse about their genitals. The more FGCS is normalised, the greater the industry's capacity to harm women and girls. Structural changes to the genitals do not materialise by magic, however strong the desire. Sensitive flesh without disease is subjected to invasive cutting and manipulating with unknown long-term effects. Given the law on FGM in many countries, legal changes are required to address the inconsistencies in genital cutting (Chapter 7). However, the relevant public bodies should not wait passively for these changes. Rather, they should take seriously the concerns raised by women's health advocates and campaigners about the social harm of FGCS (Chapter 10) and act decisively to limit the potential for harm. They could (1) introduce an ethically and psychosocially informed process of accountability that is mandatory for all registered providers; (2) stipulate strict advertising standards; (3) debunk rather than submit to the myths of choice and self-improvement in policy and guidance documents; and (4) facilitate critical conversations between relevant academic and professional disciplines, and make these conversations accessible to lay audiences. These are the least changes that women and girls like Madison, Kate and Nevaeh should be able to count on.

References

1. Parekh B. *Rethinking multiculturalism: Cultural diversity and political theory.* Cambridge, MA: Harvard University Press; 2000, p. 275.

2. Johnsdotter S, Essén B. Genitals and ethnicity: The politics of genital modifications. *Reprod Health Matters.* 2010 May;18(35):29–37. doi: 10.1016/S0968-8080(10)35495-4.

3. Liao LM, Creighton SM. Requests for cosmetic genitoplasty: How should health care providers respond? *BMJ.* 2007;334:1090–2.

4. Conroy RM. Female genital mutilation: Whose problem, whose solution? *BMJ.* 2006; 333:106–7.

5. Braun V. In search of (better) sexual pleasure: Female genital 'cosmetic' surgery. *Sexualities.* 2005;8:407–24.

6. International Society of Aesthetic Plastic Surgery (ISAPS). Global Statistics 2016. Available from: www.isaps.org/medical-professionals/isaps-global-statistics/

7. All India Congress of Obstetrics and Gynaecology 2018. Available from: www.aicog2018.org/image/Pro_Aesthetic%20Gynaecology.pdf

8. Crouch NS, Dean R, Michala L, Liao L-M, Creighton SM. Clinical characteristics of women and girls seeking labia reduction surgery. *BJOG.* 2011;118:1507–10. doi:10.1111/j1471-0528.2011.03088.

9. Tiefer L. Female cosmetic genital surgery: Freakish or inevitable? Analysis from medical marketing, bioethics and feminist theory. *Feminism Psychol.* 2008;18:466–79.

10. Smail, D. *Power, interest and psychology: Elements of a social materialist understanding of distress.* Monmouth, UK: PCCS Books; 2010.

11. Liao LM, Wood D, Creighton SM. Between a rock and a hard place: Parents choosing normalising cosmetic genital surgery for their children. *BMJ.* 2015;351:h5124.

12. Conn JJ, Jacobs HS. Managing hirsuitism in gynaecological practice. *BJOG.* 1998; 105:687–96.

13. Keegan A, Liao LM, Boyle M. Hirsuitism: A psychological analysis. *J Health Psychol.* 2003;8(3):327–45.

14. NHS Choices. What is gynaecomastia? Available from: www.nhs.uk/chq/Pages/885.aspx?CategoryID=61

15. Jain R. Muscle or man-boobs? Available from: http://riverbanksclinic.co.uk/cosmetic-surgery/gynecomastia/muscle-or-man-boobs/

16. American Society of Plastic Surgeons. 2017 Plastic surgery statistics. Available from: www.plasticsurgery.org/news/plastic-surgery-statistics

17. Krakovsky AA. State of the art in phalloplasty. *Am J Cosmetic Surg.* 2005;22(3):172–8.

18. Bramwell R. Invisible labia: The representation of female external genitals in women's magazines. *Sex Relat Ther.* 2002;17:187–90.

19. Kleck RE, Strenta, A. Perceptions of the impact of negatively valued physical characteristics on social interaction. *J Personality Social Psychol.* 1980; 39(5): 861–73.

20. Smolak L. Body Image. In: Worell J, Goodheart, CD (eds), *Handbook of girls' and women's psychological health: Gender and well-being across the lifespan.* Oxford Series in Clinical Psychology. New York: Oxford University Press; 2006, pp. 69–76.

21. Braun V, Wilkinson S. Socio-cultural representations of the vagina. *J Reprod Inf Psychol.* 2001;9(1):17–32.

22. Dolezal L. *The body and shame: Phenomenology, feminism and the socially shaped body.* Lanham, MD: Lexington; 2015, p. 132.

23. Streuli JC, Vayena E, Cavicchia-Balmer Y, Huber J. Shaping parents: Impact of contrasting professional counselling on parents' decision making for children with disorders of sex development. *J Sex Med.* 2013;10(8):1953–60.

24. BBC News. PIP breast implants health scare. Available from: www.bbc.co.uk/news/health-16391522

25. Department of Health. Review of the regulation of cosmetic interventions. 2013. Available from: www.gov.uk/government/uploads/system/uploads/attachment_data/file/192028/Review_of_the_Regulation_of_Cosmetic_Interventions.pdf

26. Society of Obstetricians and Gynaecologists of Canada. Female genital cosmetic surgery. *J Obstet Gynaecol Can* 2013; 35(12):e1–e5.

27. Royal College of Obstetricians and Gynaecologists. Ethical considerations in relation to female genital cosmetic surgery (FGCS). 2013. Available from: www.rcog.org.uk/globalassets/documents/guidelines/ethics-issues-and-resources/rcog-fgcs-ethical-opinion-paper.pdf

28. British Society for Paediatric and Adolescent Gynaecology. Labial reduction surgery (labiaplasty) on adolescents. 2013. Available from: www.britspag.org/sites/default/files/downloads/Labiaplasty%20%20final%20Position%20Statement.pdf

29. Learner H, Rundell C, Liao LM, Creighton SM. Botched labiaplasty: Online promotion of revision labiaplasty. Abstract at the British Society for Paediatric and Adolescent Gynaecology Annual Meeting, London UK, March 2018.

30. Goodman M. Revisions, redoes, and botched genital plastic surgery. Available from: www .drmichaelgoodman.com/revisions-redos-and-bot ched-genital-plastic-surgery

31. General Medical Council. Consent: Patients and doctors making decisions together. 2008. Available from: www.gmc-uk.org/guidance/ethical_guidance/co nsent_guidance_index.asp

32. Liao LM, Chadwick PM, Tamar-Mattis A. Informed consent in pediatric and adolescent gynaecological practice: From ethical principles to ethical behaviours. In Creighton SM, Balen A, Breech L, Liao L-M (eds), *Pediatric and adolescent gynecology: A problem based approach.* Cambridge: Cambridge University Press; 2018, pp. 45–52.

Female Genital Anatomy

Naomi S. Crouch

Introduction

The vulva is a poorly described and understood part of a woman's body. Part of this may reflect historical social construct: the dictionary definition of male genital anatomy describes the function and action of the organs while the corresponding definition for female genital anatomy refers to the location only.

This chapter describes the anatomy, physiology and function of the vulva and then considers where this is placed within the general understanding of women and the medical community.

Anatomy

The vulva can be considered to be the area bordered by the mons pubis at the base of the abdomen, the anus and the folds of the thighs on either side. Contained within this area are the labia majora, and labia minora which borders the central vaginal opening, known as the introitus, and the urethral opening or meatus. The clitoris sits in the midline above the urethral meatus. The area between the vaginal introitus and anus is known as the perineum and is the meeting point of several pelvic floor muscles.

To understand the anatomy and function of the vulva in adulthood it is useful to revisit the embryological development of this area. While genetic sex is determined at conception, development of the genital area into a typical female or male system does not take place until around 8 weeks of embryonic life. This is triggered by the sex-determining region of the Y chromosome (*SRY*) gene, which leads a cascade of events resulting in genital development.

Internal Genital Development

The genital duct system, which in adult females comprises the uterus and Fallopian tubes, and the vagina, consists of the Müllerian duct (MD) and the Woolfian duct (WD) systems. These are each a set of paired

tubes and are precursors of the female and male internal genital anatomy respectively. Both coexist initially in all fetuses, until the action of the *SRY* gene on the developing testes leads to expression of anti-Müllerian hormone (AMH), resulting in repression of the MD with only the WD remaining. This then allows the male genital internal anatomy to develop, with regression of the MD and any potential female structures. This usually takes place between 7 and 8 weeks of fetal life. However, in the absence of AMH the MD will persist and proliferate in the female fetus, proceeding to form the internal structures typically seen in females, at around 8–9 weeks.

The two MD tubes join in the midline, with the internal walls at the points of contact dissolving, forming the uterus, cervix and upper two-thirds of the vagina. The free ends at the top of the tubes proceed to form the Fallopian tubes. The ovaries form separately from the MD, on the gonadal ridge near the diaphragm. They descend towards the pelvis, finally lying adjacent to the Fallopian tubes on the pelvic side wall.

The External Genitalia and Urinary Opening

The vulva develops from a membrane and fold between the legs known as the cloacal membrane and cloacal fold. These proceed to form a bud in the midline, known as the central genital tubercle with paired folds and swellings lying on either side of the midline. These differentiate into the clitoris, the labia majora and the labia minora respectively. The labia majora appear flattened and the labia minora are tiny folds of skin on either side of the midline. The clitoris itself develops two paired corporal bodies which meet at the clitoral glans, at the tip of the clitoris. The glans has a covering of skin, the clitoral hood, which runs down to meet the labia minora on either side. The clitoral hood is derived from a layer of cells which develops at the top of the clitoris. Further genital and anal folds also develop, resulting in

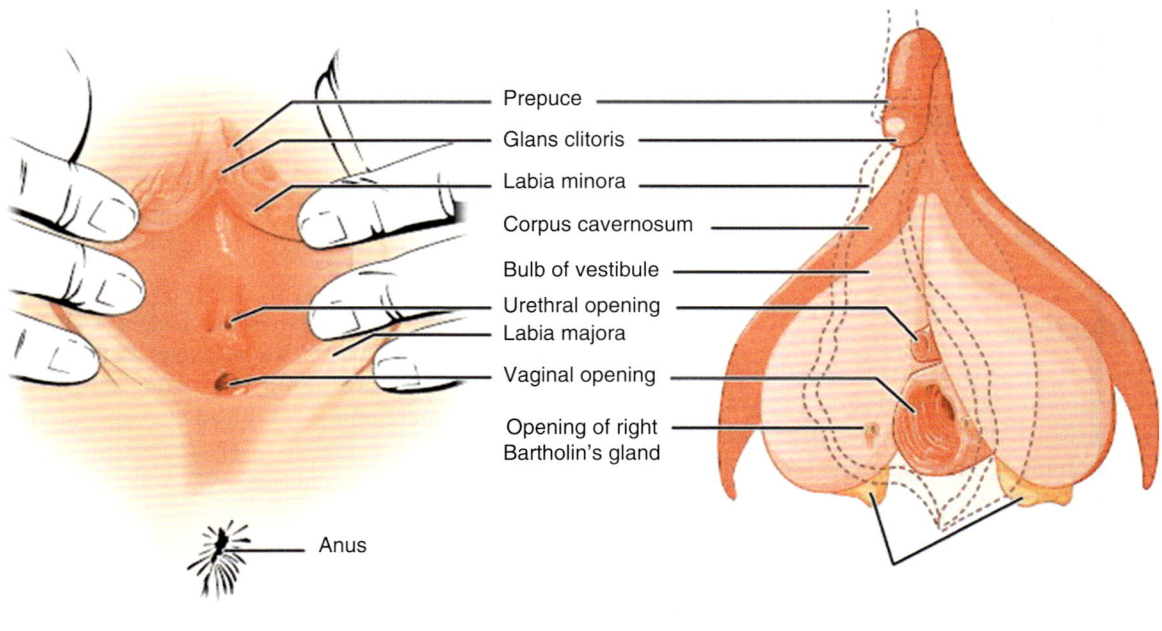

Vulva: External anterior view

Vulva: Internal anteriolateral view

Prepuce
Glans clitoris
Labia minora
Corpus cavernosum
Bulb of vestibule
Urethral opening
Labia majora
Vaginal opening
Opening of right Bartholin's gland
Anus

Figure 2.1 The vulva showing the urethra, vagina and anus, and the internal view with the clitoris and accessory glands.

a separation between the anus and combined urethral and vaginal opening, which further divides into the urethra and the vagina. This sequence of events results in the usual three separate openings onto the female genital area (see Figure 2.1).

The lower third of the vagina moves upwards to join the upper vagina, followed by dissolution of the meeting point, allowing the vagina to become a continuous tube leaving just the circumference behind, which is the hymen.

By 20 weeks of gestation, the female genitalia are developed [1].

Variations of Fetal Vulval Development

Male external genital development is mediated by androgen hormones, including testosterone expressed from the developing testes, which act upon the androgen receptor (AR), resulting in development of the central genital tubercle into a penis enclosing the urethra, and changing the genital folds into the scrotum. The testes pass through from the abdomen down into the scrotum.

A female fetus therefore can develop a more typically male appearance if higher than usual levels of androgen hormone are expressed. This leads to enlargement of the clitoris and lack of complete separation of the urethra

and vagina, resulting in only one opening to the outside rather than the more usual two. Conversely, a lack of typical male development may occur if androgen hormones are not expressed or recognised by the developing genetic male fetus. Interestingly, there appears to be a continuum in anatomical development between the level of androgen hormone and the distance between the base of the clitoris and the female urethra. Females who are least able to recognise androgen hormones develop a longer distance between the clitoris and the urethra, whereas those with a higher level of hormones will have a urethra which opens very close to the clitoris [2].

This therefore illustrates how females with increased androgen hormones during pregnancy will develop a uterus and vagina, as determined by the absence of the *SRY* gene, but also enlargement of the clitoris due to the action of androgens on the central genital tubercle. Where this is very marked, babies may be mistakenly assigned male sex, with the clitoris appearing to look like a penis, and only later presenting with a salt-wasting crisis characteristic of congenital adrenal hyperplasia.

For those with a Y chromosome, if the gonads (future ovaries or testes) have not developed in the usual way and are non-functional, no response can be mounted to the *SRY* gene and therefore AMH will not be expressed. This allows the development of the MD, regression of the WD and results in internal typically female structures. Similarly, such gonads will be unable to express androgens and therefore also unable to promote a typical male external genital appearance, leading to a female appearance externally. This would result in the birth of a baby girl who has XY chromosomes.

Development during Childhood and Adolescence

The genital tract remains essentially quiescent from birth and during early childhood. The effect of maternal oestrogen slowly decreases for approximately 6 months after birth. Occasionally an infant may have a small uterine bleed as a withdrawal bleed while the effects of maternal oestrogen wear off. For those who are born preterm, an isolated clitoromegaly may be observed and will persist throughout childhood [3]. Once any other causes for this have been excluded, parents can be reassured that this is a variant of normality and no treatment is indicated.

During childhood the labia minora remain very thin and small, and the vulva generally has a flattened appearance. With the onset of the first hormonal signals coming from the brain to the ovaries gradual changes to the genital tissues occur. These hormonal pulses start from age 8 onwards, and slowly increase in size and frequency. The action of androgens on the tissues results in pubic hair developing over the mons and labia majora. The labia minora elongate and darken in colour, and usually protrude beyond the labia majora. The mons pubis and the labia majora slowly develop fat pads. The clitoris enlarges with further development of the paired corpora, which run for several centimetres inside the pelvic bone, at the pubic rami. The clitoral glans enlarges and is covered by the developing clitoral hood, which becomes more prominent while running on to meet the labia minora.

The vulva takes many years to develop fully. Changes in the labia minora are often observed first, along with pubic hair development, as a result of the effect of androgen hormone. The labia majora fat pads may take many years to develop fully, leading to a relative prominence of labia minora as part of the appearance of the vulva. Tanner described pubic hair development, which is still used today as a means to gauge pubertal development [4]. However, labial anatomy has never been described in detail throughout puberty in the manner of breast development, limiting knowledge regarding normal pubertal development [5].

One study assessed genital dimensions in prepubertal children from 1 month to 10 years, and developed algorithms to predict expected measurements according to age, weight and height [6]. For older children, significant variation continues to be seen in the external anatomy [7] (see Figure 2.2). A study assessed 58 girls and observed a linear relationship between age and genital dimensions. The clitoral hood was noted to be a separate structure from the labia minora in all age groups, reflecting its embryological origins. A variety of shapes were noted, being variously described as a horseshoe, trumpet, coffee bean or tent. All of these papers illustrated wide diversity in genital dimensions, yet the information is promoted as having applicability for those seeking to alter the vulval area for cosmetic reasons [6].

The Adult Vulva

Once fully developed, the adult vulva consists of the mons pubis, which leads to the labia majora on either side of the vaginal introitus. Situated laterally on each side of the introitus are the labia minora. The labia majora consists of hair-bearing skin, and androgens will promote growth of darker and coarser pubic hair. This will grow up to the labia minora, which have a mucosal surface on both sides. Pubic hair also extends over the mons pubis and often onto the top of the thighs. The labia minora vary in appearance but tend to have a rugose texture and are darker than the surrounding tissue. A wide variety of dimensions have been described in the literature, but it is not unusual for labial width to measure up to 5 cm at the widest part, and sometimes beyond [8]. It is also common and usual for the labia minora to protrude beyond the labia majora, which is not necessarily understood by girls and women [5].

Surrounding the vaginal introitus and urethra are various glands, often known as Skene's glands, Bartholin's glands and vestibular glands. Skene's glands are situated just laterally to the urethral meatus, with Bartholin's glands being placed at 5 and 7 o'clock on the vaginal introitus. The glands of the vestibule occur at various positions around the introitus, just up to the level of the hymen. The clitoris is situated approximately 3 cm above the urethral meatus, which is tucked just on the anterior vaginal wall [8]. The blood supply to the vulva is derived mainly from

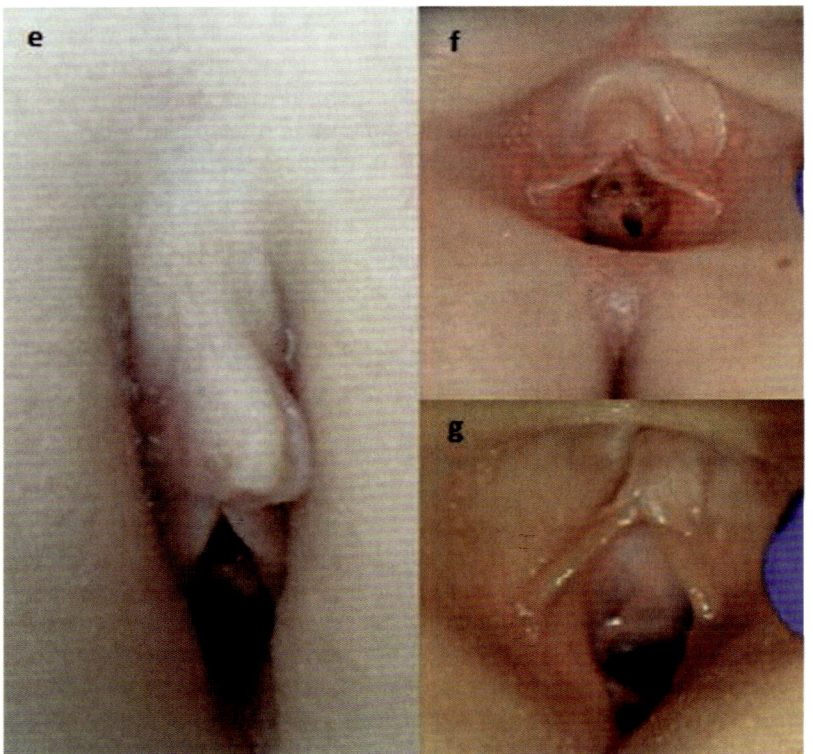

Figure 2.2 Study of clitoral hood anatomy in the pediatric population. (From Brodie KE, Grantham EC, Huguelet PS, Caldwell BT, Westfall NJ, Wilcox DT. *J Pediatr Urol.* 2016 Jun;12(3):177.e1-5. Reproduced with permission from Elsevier.)

the pudendal artery, with the inferior epigastric artery supplying the mons pubis. The innervation to the vulva and its component parts is largely supplied by the pudendal nerve, arising from S2–4, although the ilioinguinal nerve (L1) and the genital branch of the genitofemoral nerve (L1–2) provide sensation to medial and lateral vulval skin.

The adult clitoris can reasonably be considered as an iceberg, with only the tip being visible. The external portion consists of paired corpora which contain erectile tissue, capped at the end by the clitoral glans. The clitoral hood covers the glans, and is more retractile than in childhood. It proceeds to meet the labia minora at the clitoral frenulum, at an angle clearly defining the start of the labia. The external clitoral body measures 2–4 cm in length and divides into two internal crura just under the pubic arch. Internally these extend laterally and inferiorly, running along the inferior pubic rami, with the crura extending for up to 9 cm (see Figure 2.1). Coursing underneath, two suspensory ligaments extend to join the mons pubis. A deeper ligament

complex extends from the symphysis pubis to join the body and bulbs of the clitoris. When described, these ligaments were found to be considerably larger than had previously been documented, and differed in shape, extent and orientation from any analogous structures in the penis [9]. The nerve supply to the clitoris is derived from the pelvic, pudendal and hypogastric nerves, with the clitoral nerve running along the inferior pubic rami accompanying the crura of the clitoris. The nerves fan out around the clitoral glans, and perforate the covering tunica of the corpora.

Postmenopausal Changes

The average age at menopause in the United Kingdom is 51, with a range of 45–55 years. Vulval changes after this time reflect waning oestrogen levels, and include a loss of labial fat pads and a gradual sparseness of pubic hair. The labia minora will experience thinning and will decrease in size with loss of architecture and detail [10]. The vagina is shortened and appears pale due to a reduction in vaginal epithelial layers. The vaginal mucosa can become dry and have a reduced response in producing lubrication during sexual activity. Many of these changes can be mediated by the use of topical oestrogen.

Physiology

The development of the whole genital area during fetal life, with an upper uterus and vaginal section descending to meet the external developing vulva, is reflected in the subsequent adult functioning of the female genital tract. Generally speaking, the upper genital tract, including the upper two-thirds of the vagina, is more concerned with reproductive function, whereas the lower and external parts are associated with sensation and sexual pleasure.

The clitoris and labia minora are rich in innervation and blood supply and contain erectile tissue, all of which are of prime importance in sexual sensation and contribution to orgasm.

The clitoris itself is a dynamic organ which becomes engorged with blood during sexual arousal. Paired clitoral arteries supply blood to the glans, with cavernosa vessels supplying the corporal system. During arousal the cavernosa fill with blood, with venous valves closing, thereby preventing drainage and facilitating erection, contributing to sexual pleasure and achievement of orgasm. After orgasm the valves open, allowing the venous flow to return to the internal pudendal vein.

The labia minora contain erectile tissue which also becomes engorged with blood during sexual arousal. Oestrogen receptors have been demonstrated on the labia minora along the free edges [10]. One study assessed 62 women and asked them to rate various parts of the vulval area on the basis of anatomy and sexual sensitivity [11]. The majority of women rated the labia minora and majora as average-sized, with 13% rating the labia as large and 5% as small. Sensitivity for the labia increased towards the vagina, with the medial edge of the labia minora being the most sensitive area. Sensitivity did not vary according to self-reported size, although those with larger labia reported higher ratings for sexual pleasure. It may be that as more erectile tissue was present, more stimulation resulted in higher levels of sexual pleasure.

In contrast to the clitoris and labia minora, the labia majora become thinner during sexual arousal, which opens the introital area and thereby promotes vaginal penetration. The accessory glands of the vulva contribute to sexual function by producing fluid during arousal and aiding lubrication for penetrative intercourse.

During sexual activity and arousal, the vagina lengthens and expands around the cervix to provide a receptacle for sperm, facilitating passage through the cervical canal and onto the Fallopian tubes with anticipated reproductive consequences. Magnetic resonance imaging (MRI) has shown that the vaginal walls enlarge with fluid during penetrative intercourse, with the anterior vaginal wall lengthening and the uterus being elevated [12]. This may contribute to positioning the cervix more closely to the posterior fornix where sperm may be deposited.

There is no evidence for the existence of the Grafenberg spot (G-spot), which was thought to be a distinct structure intimately related to sexual pleasure and situated on the anterior vaginal wall. It is more likely that any increased sexual sensation is related to clitoral fibres around the urethra. Female ejaculation is also not consistently described; where it occurs it may be related to fluid being expressed from paraurethral (Skene's) glands on either side of the urethra.

Clitoral surgery is known to risk sexual function and achievement of orgasm. Work assessing long-term outcome of childhood feminising surgery for those born with disorders/difference of sex development (intersex) showed a 1:4 anorgasmia rate for women who had undergone surgery [13]. Clitoral sensation is impaired in those who have undergone surgery [14]. Given the anatomical distribution of nerves, and the inevitability of surgical incisions causing cutting of nerve fibres in a densely innervated structure, it is likely that repeated surgery would risk function further.

Recent work assessed women who had undergone female genital cutting of the clitoris and compared them with unaffected women matched for age and parity [15]. Those who had undergone cutting had a significantly smaller clitoral volume and also reported significantly lower scores on sexual function and desire. Interestingly, there was no difference on the subscores of orgasm desire and satisfaction, but those who had undergone cutting did report significantly more dyspareunia.

Standardising the Vulva?

An emerging and increasing interest in 'normalising' female genital anatomy has highlighted the lack of accurate information on typical genital dimensions.

Such information may be utilised by those performing feminising surgery for those born with atypical genitalia, or by well women seeking female genital cosmetic surgery (FGCS). In contrast to descriptions of male anatomy, information in the medical literature is sparse. One study assessed 50 premenopausal women who had not undergone surgery, nor expressed concern about anatomical appearance, and demonstrated a wide range of measurements, in particular for the clitoris and the labia minora [8]. This has been widely used as a reference text, and others have replicated its findings.

Vulval anatomy appears to have ratios, which may be related to relative androgenisation of the area. One article related this to an 'Androgen Index', where the size of the clitoris was inversely related to clitoral-to-urethral distance [2]. Therefore, altering one part of the vulva may change this ratio, and potentially perceived satisfaction with appearance.

A more recent study assessed the anatomical dimensions of 32 women and compared this with a validated sexual function tool [16]. Again, wide variability in the range of measurements was observed. No difference was observed in the achievement of orgasm, or not, and any of the genital dimensions measured, suggesting that vulval dimensions per se are not related to sexual function or satisfaction.

Medical Representation

The vulva has proved to be a contentious area in terms of anatomical description. Human anatomy could reasonably be considered as unchanging and fixed, yet descriptions of the vulval area and the clitoris in particular have varied considerably over the years.

In 1844 the anatomist Georg Ludwig Kobelt published an essay on clitoral anatomy with highly detailed drawings accompanying the area [17]. The clitoris was identified as having a shaft, glans, bulbs and associated muscles. He also commented on the significant nerve bundle and blood supply, noting the paired dorsal clitoral arteries.

Such pioneering work, however, was not replicated in subsequent anatomy textbooks. Indeed the vulva and clitoris have decreased in size over time. *Grey's Anatomy* is a famous textbook which has been published for more than 150 years, yet variations in vulval anatomy are seen in different editions. The 1901 edition shows the clitoris to be a fairly prominent structure, with labels to the prepuce,

glans and body of the clitoris (see Figure 2.3)[18]. The 1918 edition, however, shows the structure as proportionately smaller compared with the rest of the vulva and with one label indicating 'clitoris' only (see Figure 2.4) [19].

More modern textbooks do not fare better. Generally male genital anatomy is presented first, with lengthy descriptions, only then followed by female anatomy, which is frequently described as being a homologue of male genital structures. The text and accompanying illustrations are also less detailed. One study assessed 30 anatomy and 29 gynaecology textbooks published between 1990 and 2011 for dimensions of the vagina, clitoris, labia

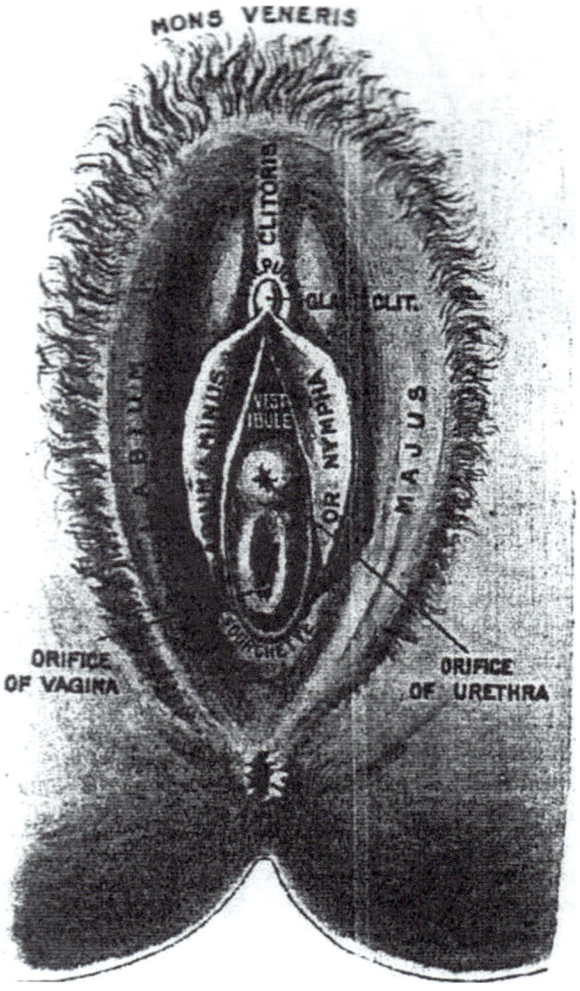

Figure 2.3 Diagram of vulval anatomy from Grays' Anatomy 1901 Edition

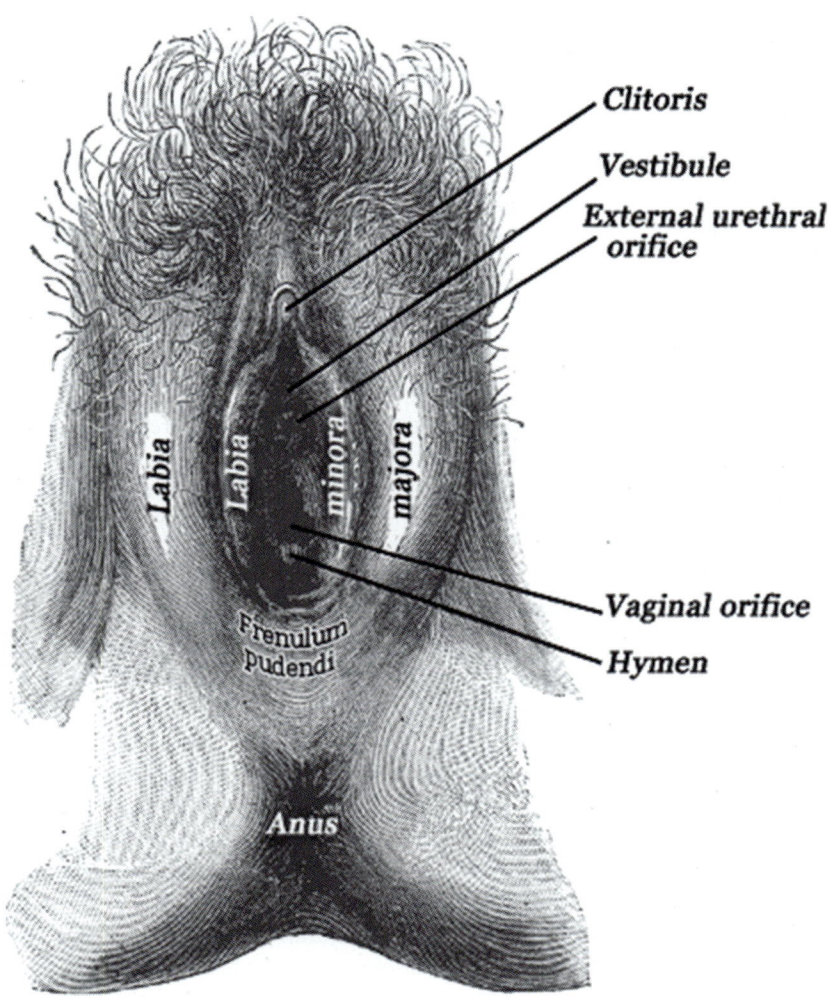

Clitoris

Vestibule

External urethral orifice

Labia

Labia

minora

majora

Frenulum pudendi

Vaginal orifice

Hymen

Anus

Figure 2.4 Diagram of vulval anatomy from Grays' Anatomy 1918 Edition

minora and majora and the number and type of illustrations [20]. None of the anatomy textbooks provided measurements for the labia, although three gynaecology textbooks did so. Only two texts gave any measurements for the labia minora, and these were noted to be considerably smaller than those in contemporaneously published medical literature. Eight texts had no illustrations or images, 5 utilised a photograph of the vulva, and 46 used the same line drawing of the external genitalia. Strikingly, no text had more than one illustration. No comment was made in any text regarding the variability of vulval anatomy in healthy women.

One possible reason for the sparseness of information could be the reliance of anatomical descriptions on cadaveric studies. Pioneering work considered that the majority of this information was derived from postmenopausal women [21], leading to an underestimation of normal dimensions. Work from the same group has continued to identify new structures, with recommendations for change in terminology in light of the new findings [22]. Different imaging modalities have identified a united complex comprising the clitoris, urethra and distal vagina, which is the locus of female sexual activity, with the proposal that this considered the clitoral complex.

To challenge the traditional and inaccurate representation of female genital anatomy, an alternative textbook was published, to present women's anatomy first and with new and detailed drawings [23].

An updated version in 1991 also included photographs of women from different ethnic groups [24].

Modern Challenges

Since the start of the new millennium, the vulva can be considered to have emerged into greater prominence in popular culture. Television shows have promoted engagement with the vulva by trends designed to draw attention to the area, such as Vajazzle. In Western culture the majority of young women are likely to prefer removing pubic hair, in contrast to older generations, leading to a high level of physical engagement with their own bodies on a regular basis. However, this may not be matched by an equal understanding and appreciation of genital anatomy and knowledge of the wide range of variation in vulval dimensions in healthy women.

Perception of Vulval Anatomy

Perception of Women

Anatomical understanding of female genital anatomy can vary among women. Not least, this is illustrated in the popular use of anatomical terms, with vagina frequently being used to describe the vulva. Misconstructions are reflected in popular catchphrases such as 'designer vagina', referring to FGCS on the vulva to change the appearance of the external genital area, rather than any surgery to the vagina, which is an internal structure.

Vulval physiology, and sexual function and pleasure in particular, are often misrepresented in popular culture such as films. In particular, female orgasm is often portrayed as achieved solely through penetrative vaginal intercourse, which would not be typical for the majority of women.

The vulva area is seen to be important to women, but one study suggested this pertains more to appearance and less to function [25]. A large study assessed 482 women to investigate common beliefs and attitudes regarding the labia minora [26]. The majority were female medical students, and the study also included 88 patients invited from outpatient clinics, divided between public and private health care settings. Ninety-five per cent of participants frequently examined the labia minora, and nearly all were aware of the concept of labial surgery to alter and reduce their appearance. Almost half believed appearance to be important, with 14% having received either positive or negative comments from a partner. Fourteen per cent also considered the appearance was abnormal, with half of those having considered surgery. What is particularly striking is the fact that the majority of participants had a high level of education and easier access than most to medical resources for information. It could be that this represents a younger population, but other work including both pre- and postmenopausal women showed that age did not affect the perception of normal anatomy [27].

One study assessed 16 adolescents who were requesting assessment of their genitalia or labia [5]. For six girls the concern was a difference in size between the labia minora. For the remainder, the issue was the width of the labia minora. A significant belief was that the labia minora were abnormal as they protruded through the labia majora. This belief was occasionally also shared by the parents.

Perception of Clinicians

Women who request FGCS will be initially assessed by a doctor. In most publicly funded health care systems this would be a general practitioner (GP) before referral to a surgeon would be considered and arranged. Referral would therefore be based on clinician assessment and opinion as to the suitability of considering a surgical procedure.

A study in London assessed reasons for the initial referral to a gynaecologist and found that one in four GP letters would use pejorative language when describing the labia minora [28]. This had the effect of reinforcing the sense of an 'abnormality' to the patient, which needed to be 'corrected'. While a few letters would ask for assessment or even reassurance for the patient, the majority were seeking surgery as a solution to the perceived issue. All women were found to have normal labia when assessed by a gynaecologist.

A small study reviewed 16 girls who were concerned about the genital area and found that 4 were referred by clinicians who described their labia as 'hypertrophied', despite having a normal assessment in clinic [5].

GPs are therefore often asked to give opinions and information on women seeking information regarding vulval anatomy, and making a decision regarding arranging an onward referral. One study examined the knowledge and attitude of more than 400 GPs regarding women requesting guidance on and referral for FGCS [29]. Strikingly, 35% had seen women under the age of 18 requesting surgery. Seventy-five per cent felt they did not have adequate knowledge of FGCS, or confidence in discussing the long-term risks of surgery. The majority felt that psychological problems underpinned the request. Of note, the survey population comprised GPs primarily with an interest in women's health and with more than 20 years of experience in general practice, yet were clearly experiencing a marked increase in this area of clinical practice to which they felt underprepared in responding.

The majority of requests for FGCS will be met in the private health care sector, where women may not necessarily require a referral from a GP. They will, however, be seen by a clinician and an opinion will be expressed as to the appropriateness of a surgical procedure. In the absence of any information regarding 'normality' a plan for surgery is therefore likely to be highly dependent on a subjective clinical opinion.

One study assessed the attitudes of 80 GPs, 43 plastic surgeons and 41 gynaecologists regarding the appearance of the vulval area and the willingness to offer surgery [30]. Plastic surgeons were more likely to favour very small labia minora as being close to the ideal, compared with GPs and gynaecologists. Two-thirds of GPs would refer a woman for surgery without any physical symptoms. Plastic surgeons were consistently more likely to offer surgery to women compared with gynaecologists, and male physicians were also significantly more likely to operate than their female colleagues.

Perception of Male Partners

It has been postulated that for women who have sex with men, their partner's opinion regarding vulval anatomy may be a significant influence in leading to requests for FGCS. One article surveyed 2,403 men on vulvar appearance, knowledge of female anatomy and opinions and awareness of FGCS [31]. The majority of men self-rated as either somewhat or very familiar with female anatomy and were able to label the anatomy correctly. Half of the sample had heard of FGCS but 75% would not encourage their partner to seek surgery to alter genital appearance. Fifty-one per cent felt the appearance of the genital area, including hair pattern, would influence them in engaging in sexual activity, but 60% stated the size of a women's labia did not affect pleasure with sexual activity. In addition, those men who had experienced more lifetime partners were more likely to rate larger labia minora as more attractive. These data suggests that men do not hold strong opinions about vulval appearance in relation to desirability for sexual activity with female partners.

Seeking Accurate Representation

Lack of Information for Women

There remains a lack of information for women regarding normal vulval anatomy. Where more accurate and realistic information is available, reassurance regarding diversity seems to follow. The art world and popular culture have started exploring this further. An example can be seen in the work by Jamie McCartney entitled "The Great Wall of Vagina" [32], which is a series of large panels comprising plaster casts of vulvas. Each panel contains 40 different vulvas, and the contrast between the appearances is clear. For women who had previously expressed concern or anxiety with the appearance of their own vulva, attending the exhibition provided reassurance and a reduction in worry [33]. Other work includes that by Suzanna Scott, who uses handbags and purses turned inside out to represent the vulva and female genital anatomy as a positive way of seeing the genital area in a new light [34].

Other websites have developed that are specifically aimed at reducing concern and anxiety regarding the appearance of the vulval area [35]. The website in [35] shows images of the vulva area, both in the traditional display, but also with women standing up and perhaps therefore reproducing the only way some women see the vulva. Other resources have also been developed for women to view and download, using alternative ways of representing the vulval anatomy and discussing the variety of appearances seen in healthy women [36]. However, with adverts for cosmetic surgery providers consistently being more prominently returned on search terms, these informative websites remain difficult for women to access unless specifically signposted.

Pathologisation of the Vulva

Female Genital Cosmetic Surgery

Increasingly well women are seeking surgical alteration of the vulva, with large increases noted since the start of the new millennium; a fivefold increase was seen in the United Kingdom between 2001 and 2010, a tripling between 2000 and 2011 in Australia and a 44% increase between 2013 and 2014 in the USA [25, 38]. These data represent the publicly funded health care systems; the majority of requests are likely to be met within private health care and no reliable data on these is available.

Most of the surgery performed is a reduction in the size of the labia minora, but requests for alteration to the clitoral hood or liposuction to the labia minora or mons pubis have also been described.

Reasons for the increase in desire for surgery are unclear but a request to alleviate physical symptoms is often presented as a significant indication [38]. There is a suggestion that women may promote symptoms which they believe health care providers may wish to hear in order to justify a referral for surgical alteration of the labia. However, on asking women directly what is hoped to be achieved by surgery, relief of symptoms is often under-represented compared with an aim of altering the appearance of the area [37].

It could be considered that requests from surgery result from more awareness of an abnormality. However, there is no evidence of an increase in labial pathology, nor a change in surgical technique, suggesting instead requests for intervention are driven by societal influences.

Normality or Abnormality?

One potential reason for the rise in FGCS could simply be the normalisation and increased societal acceptance of surgery as providing a solution to a perceived problem. Increasingly the internet is used as an important tool for those considering cosmetic surgery. Michala et al. found that this was the primary source of information for older adolescents seeking labiaplasty [5]. A study in the Netherlands showed that women who had used the internet to access information were more likely to view surgery as acceptable, compared with those who had sought information from mainstream media, peers or a clinician [26]. A further literature review and qualitative analysis identified five themes as contributing to the normalisation of FGCS [39]. These were pathologisation of genital diversity; female genital appearance as being important for well-being; characteristics of women's genitals as important for their sex life; the female body as degenerative and improvable through surgery; and FGCS as being safe, easy and effective.

The pathologisation of genital diversity extends to the medical literature. Labial hypertrophy is a phrase which is commonly used and which sounds reassuringly medical, yet lacks any definition or validation. Information is available regarding the normal limits of the labia minora, yet these are made with no reference to the height or body mass index of the woman [33]. There are also repeated references made to enlarged labia, which

apparently cause problems for women, with no definition of what 'enlarged' may be considered to be.

With increasing knowledge of the anatomy and physiology of the labia minora, coupled with concern about pathologisation of the vulva, some studies have sought to reassure that surgery is straightforward and risk-free. A recent study was based on four cadaveric samples and assessed nerve density in portions of the labia [40], although this does not assess the physiology and erectile component of the structure. There are also no controlled post-operative studies available of sexual function and satisfaction in women who have undergone such surgical procedures.

Labial reduction surgery remains an unproven treatment for an unidentified pathology, which appears to be driven by societal desirability for a particular prepubertal 'Barbie doll' appearance of the adult vulva.

Conclusion

The vulva is a complex structure which is active and dynamic during sexual activity. Vulval anatomy is poorly understood and described in medical textbooks, and the representation of this has varied over time. The vulva takes many years to develop fully and changes significantly over a woman's lifetime. An accurate and realistic representation in an internet age remains surprisingly scarce, and is not keeping pace with cultural interest in the vulval area, in particular labial anatomy.

Future work is aimed at redressing this balance, with the development of educational resources available to women and clinicians. Clear and unambiguous messages regarding the normality and variance in vulval anatomy are needed from medical literature and clinicians. Without this women will continue to struggle to find reliable information about this hidden part of a woman's anatomy.

References

1. Sajjad Y. Development of the genital ducts and external genitalia in the early human embryo. *J Obstet Gynaecol Res*. 2010;36(5):929–37.

2. Crouch NS, Michala L, Creighton SM, Conway GS. Androgen-dependent measurements of female genitalia in women with complete androgen insensitivity syndrome. *BJOG* 2011;118(1):84–7. doi: 10.1111/j.1471–0528.2010.02778.x.

3. Williams CE, Nakhal RS, Achermann JC, Creighton SM. Persistent unexplained congenital clitoromegaly in

females born extremely prematurely. *J Pediatr Urol.* 2013;9(6 Pt A):962–5.

4. Marshall WA, Tanner JM. Variations in pattern of pubertal changes in girls. *Arch Dis Child.* 1969;44 (235):291–303.

5. Michala L, Koliantzaki S, Antsaklis A. Protruding labia minora: Abnormal or just uncool? *J Psychosom Obstet Gynaecol.* 2011;32(3):154–6.

6. Akbiyik F, Kutlu AO. External genital proportions in prepubertal girls: A morphometric reference for female genitoplasty. *J Urol.* 2010;184(4):1476–81.

7. Brodie KE, Grantham EC, Huguelet PS, Caldwell BT, Westfall NJ, Wilcox DT. Study of clitoral hood anatomy in the pediatric population. *J Pediatr Urol.* 2016;12(3):177.e1–5. doi: 10.1016/j.jpurol.2015.12.006.

8. Lloyd J, Crouch NS, Minto CL, Liao LM, Creighton SM. Female genital appearance: "Normality" unfolds. *BJOG.* 2005;112(5):643–6.

9. Rees MA, O'Connell HE, Plenter RJ, Hutson JM. The suspensory ligament of the clitoris: Connective tissue supports of the erectile tissues of the female urogenital region. *Clin Anat.* 2000;13(6):397–403.

10. Martin-Alguacil N, Pfaff DW, Kow LM, Schober JM. Oestrogen receptors and their relation to neural receptive tissue of the labia minora. *BJU Int.* 2008;101 (11):1401–6.

11. Schober JM, Alguacil NM, Cooper RS, Pfaff DW, Meyer-Bahlburg HF. Self-assessment of anatomy, sexual sensitivity, and function of the labia and vagina. *Clin Anat.* 2015;28(3):355–62.

12. Schultz WW, van Andel P, Sabelis I, Mooyaart E. Magnetic resonance imaging of male and female genitals during coitus and female sexual arousal. *BMJ.* 1999;319(7225):1596–600.

13. Minto CL, Liao LM, Woodhouse CR, Ransley PG, Creighton SM. The effect of clitoral surgery on sexual outcome in individuals who have intersex conditions with ambiguous genitalia: A cross-sectional study. *Lancet.* 2003;361(9365):1252–7.

14. Crouch NS, Liao LM, Woodhouse CR, Conway GS, Creighton SM. Sexual function and genital sensitivity following feminizing genitoplasty for congenital adrenal hyperplasia. *J Urol.* 2008;179(2):634–8.

15. Abdulcadir J, Botsikas D, Bolmont M, et al. Sexual anatomy and function in women with and without genital mutilation: A cross-sectional study. *J Sex Med.* 2016;13(2):226–37.

16. Krissi H, Ben-Shitrit G, Aviram A, et al. Anatomical diversity of the female external genitalia and its association to sexual function. *Eur J Obstet Gynecol Reprod Biol.* 2016;196:44–7.

17. Kobelt GL. *Die mäanlichen und weibleichn Wollustorgane des Menschen und einiger Säugethiere.* Freiberg; 1844.

18. Gray H. *Anatomy: Descriptive and surgical.* London: Longmans Green and Co. 1901.

19. Gray H. *Anatomy of the human body.* Philadelphia: Lea and Febiger; 1918.

20. Andrikopoulou M, Michala L, Creighton SM, Liao LM. The normal vulva in medical textbooks. *J Obstet Gynaecol.* 2013;33(7):648–50.

21. O'Connell HE, Hutson JM, Anderson CR, Plenter RJ. Anatomical relationship between urethra and clitoris. *J Urol.* 1998;159(6):1892–7.

22. O'Connell HE, Eizenberg N, Rahman M, Cleeve J. The anatomy of the distal vagina: Towards unity. *J Sex Med.* 2008;5(8):1883–91.

23. The Federation of Feminist Women's Health Centers. *A new view of a woman's body.* Illus. Suzann Gage New York: Simon and Schuster; 1981.

24. The Federation of Feminist Women's Health Centers, *A new view of a woman's body.* Illus. Suzann Gage San Diego: Feminist Health Press; 1991.

25. Howarth C, Hayes J, Simonis M, Temple-Smith M. 'Everything's neatly tucked away': Young women's views on desirable vulval anatomy. *Cult Health Sex.* 2016;3:1–16.

26. Koning M, Zeijlmans IA, Bouman TK, van der Lei B. Female attitudes regarding labia minora appearance and reduction with consideration of media influence. *Aesthet Surg J.* 2009;29(1):65–71.

27. Yurteri-Kaplan LA, Antosh DD, Sokol AI, et al. Interest in cosmetic vulvar surgery and perception of vulvar appearance. *Am J Obstet Gynecol.* 2012;207 (5):428.e1–7.

28. Deans R, Liao LM, Crouch NS, Creighton SM. Why are women referred for female genital cosmetic surgery? *Med J Aust.* 2011;195(2):99.

29. Simonis M, Manocha R, Ong JJ. Female genital cosmetic surgery: A cross-sectional survey exploring knowledge, attitude and practice of general practitioners. *BMJ Open.* 2016;6(9):e013010.

30. Reitsma W, Mourits MJ, Koning M, Pascal A, van der Lei B. No (wo)man is an island–the influence of physicians' personal predisposition to labia minora appearance on their clinical decision making: A cross-sectional survey. *J Sex Med.* 2011;8(8):2377–85.

31. Mazloomdoost D, Crisp CC, Westermann LB, Benbouajili JM, Kleeman SD, Pauls RN. Survey of male perceptions regarding the vulva. *Am J Obstet Gynecol.* 2015;213(5):731.e1–9. doi: 10.1016/j.ajog.2015.05.063.

32. www.greatwallofvagina.co.uk

33. Clerico C, Lari A, Mojallal A, Boucher F. Anatomy and aesthetics of the labia minora: The ideal vulva? *Aesth Plast Surg.* 2017;41(3):714–19.

34. www.suzannascott.com

35. www.labiallibrary.co.au

36. www.britspag.org.uk

37. Bramwell R, Morland C, Garden AS. Expectations and experience of labial reduction: A qualitative study. *BJOG.* 2007;114(12):1493–9.

38. Mowat H, McDonald K, Dobson AS, Fisher J, Kirkman M. The contribution of online content to the promotion and normalisation of female genital cosmetic surgery: A systematic review of the literature. *BMC Womens Health.* 2015;15:110.

39. Kelishadi SS, Omar R, Herring N, et al. The safe labiaplasty: A study of nerve density in labia minora and its implications. *Aesthet Surg J.* 2016;36(6):705–9. doi: 10.1093/asj/sjw002.

Selling a Perfect Vulva? Selling a 'Normal' Vulva!

Virginia Braun

A surgeon says women are getting designer vagina surgery to look better in leggings

Let us preface this by saying that there's nothing wrong with getting labiaplasty.

It's entirely within everyone's rights to make alterations to their body for whatever reason, and many people with vaginas undergo surgery to deal with pain and discomfort caused by longer labia.

It's just a shame that there seems to be a trend for labiaplasty done purely for cosmetic reasons, to fit an ideal of what the vulva 'should' look like [1].

Such opening sentences to an article (about labiaplasty) would have been unimaginable not *that* long ago. Not anymore. For almost 20 years, the 'designer vagina' – genital cosmetic surgery for the vagina and vulva – has been part of public discourse and material practice. We now have a generation of young adults who have developed body and genital awareness, genital aesthetic preferences and indeed ideas and expectations about genito-sexuality, in a context in which surgical and non-surgical interventions to alter form and function of the vulva/vagina just are. This creates a different set of potentials, and alongside this, a different set of obligations, around the genitalia. Today, just 'taking what you are given', genitally, is not the only option available to you – it is a 'choice' that you make. Engaging in some level of aesthetic genital labour [2, 3] is now required, in Global North/Westernised nations, as well as many others globally [4].[1]

---

[1] The idea of genital alteration of girls and women (and sometimes men) is not unfamiliar around the world. Much concern had focused on 'other' countries' 'cultural traditions' around genital cutting – which have rightly been questioned on health and human rights grounds. For a discussion of the continuities and discontinuities in how we make sense of different genital cutting, through the analytic lens of reproductive justice, see [4].

Ellen Scott's article, which includes a critical or questioning voice, starts with a caveat: "There's nothing wrong with getting labiaplasty" [1]. This logic seems dominant, yet many critics would question the logic of a sentence like that. Many of us have been critical of these genital procedures (commonly referred to as female genital cosmetic surgery [FGCS]), in the academy [5–8], in popular culture [9] and through activism [10]. I have examined representation and discourse around genital cosmetic surgery, and implications of these, since the early days of the practice [2, 4, 11–17]. In contrast to the opening quote, I have argued that there is *much* that is wrong with (getting) labiaplasty. The aim of my argument is not to blame the individuals who have labiaplasty, for bad choices or some kind of false consciousness. Instead, it is to suggest that not every option of 'choice' provided is positive, and that choosing per se is not the same as liberation or bodily empowerment.

I will summarise some of the key issues in critiques of FGCS, and provide some new analysis about genital aesthetic desire. I emphasise the implications of these procedures for people with vulvo-vaginal genitalia. Even if we see the surgeries and non-surgical interventions as problematic, it is tempting to see them as *solutions* that arose in relation to a real existing problem. I will argue that offers an easy, but *inadequate*, analysis of the issue. These procedures do not simply respond to a problem; instead, representation and practice of these procedures are part of creating our socio-cultural – and thus individual – ideas about what a vulva/vagina *should be like* – and, indeed, of bigger questions about how we make sense of bodily distress, and the appropriate responses to them.

But Isn't There a Real Problem?

The short answer is yes. Women have a long history of experiencing genital distress, a history that preceded these procedures [18, 19], and has continued since they appeared. Before I discuss genital distress, however, I need to address the terms at stake: women and female genitalia. In the context of some fairly rapid shifts in understandings and categorisations of gendered identity, both terms are now understood as potentially exclusionary – people who identify as women may not have a vulva and/or a vagina; people who identify as men may have a vulva and/or a vagina. Language is problematic. The concept of 'female' genitalia cuts across a messy intersection between understandings of (biological) sex and (personal/social) gender. There is no easy definition here. Most research around 'FGCS' has focused on cisgendered women (the genital experiences and surgeries of trans [or non-binary], as well as intersex people, tends to be treated separately); the literature of genital distress I discuss focuses almost entirely on cisgendered (non-intersex) women. This reflects the scope and focus of 'FGCS': they are aimed at women, conceptualised within a sex/gender binary, women whose genitalia trouble them, but whose sex and gendered identities do not. My use of terms such as women throughout this chapter, then, reflects the scholarship, but is imperfect.

Women whose gendered bodies or identities are *not* outside binary norms experience considerable levels of genital distress, anxiety or 'dislike' [18–22]. Distress can be mild or significantly interfere with women's potential for living their lives. Anxiety and/or distress have clustered around appearance and hygiene-oriented concerns. Related to hygiene, women express concerns that their genitalia are somehow unclean, and in particular smelly or dirty. *Any* discharge – a natural physiological part of vaginal function – is sometimes treated as problematic. A multi-billion dollar industry of 'feminine hygiene products' has supported and perpetuated this perception. This industry persists despite various critiques [23], and use of the products has been associated with cleanliness and freshness [24]. In relation to appearance, women report concerns about 'messiness' and 'ugliness', and (perceived to be) large(r) labia minora, uneven labia minora, more wrinkly labia or significant colour variation can be seen as problematic. The idea that hygiene and appearance should be concerns – that the vulva is legitimately ugly, dirty, smelly – is reinforced through a plethora of sometimes humorous, sometimes hateful, slang terms which construct the vulva in these ways [25].

In all of these, the concern is as much – sometimes more – about how *another* person will perceive and judge the genitalia, than about how the individual herself feels. For instance, concern about smell or, particularly, taste, relates typically to an imagined sexual partner; visual aspects also have an element of this (which also informs pubic hair practice [26]). However, much of the framing around FGCS, through public media stories and marketing by surgeons, is almost exclusively in terms of the self – your *own* aesthetic preferences; your *own* sexual response and experience [16]. The rhetoric frames it as a practice *for the self* – an act you can choose as part of a general project of improvement of body/self. In this, FGCS aligns with the general shift towards individualised understandings of, and investment in, the self, that has been characterised as a neoliberal self-improving agent [11, 27].

What Do Women Say?

To explore labial concerns expressed 'naturalistically', I, along with Chloe Rigg and Dr Helen Madden,[2] analysed commentary from women in online sexual/health forums regarding labial appearance concerns and considerations of labiaplasty. Using Google and Yahoo (US, UK, NZ sites), we searched using "I want labiaplasty", "I hate my vagina", "I hate my labia" and "Are my labia normal?" and compiled the first 10 hits from each search. After excluding surgeon sites, professional-opinion sites and videos, the dataset comprised mostly 'naturally occurring' discussions – such as discussion forums. These offer a valuable source of 'everyday sense-making' outside the realm of researcher influence [28]. Following ethical considerations, we chose only to access open/public forum data, but do not report usernames in the analysis [28, 29]. A thematic analysis [30] identified two coexisting but contradictory patterns of meaning: the first, "the ideal vulva," captured the way an 'ideal' vulva was articulated; the second, "we can't all be Barbie," captured an acknowledged and sometimes idealised opposition between this 'ideal' and 'real life'.

The ideal vulva was expressed by people who contrasted their own vulva with public imagery:

> any time I've ever seen a vagina, be it through porn or through educational diagrams, it always looks

---

[2] Analysis was carried out by Chloe Rigg for her BA(Hons) dissertation; Helen Madden supervised the project during a time when health issues prevented my active engagement.

streamlined and 'neat'. Mine looks like old flesh that's been chewed on by a dog. I'm incredibly self-conscious about how much the inner lips stick out. I'm curious too, how many women feel this way?

(F; I hate my vagina; Yahoo UK #2)

This meaning contained two distinct ideas. First, the ideal vulva (often expressed as 'vagina') should be 'small' and 'neat' [31, 32]. Personally assessed anatomical difference from this ideal produced challenges for embodied self-acceptance: "I want to feel like it's normal but it's hard because I know that others are smaller and definitely not like mine" (A; I hate my labia; Google UK #6). This connects to Moran and Lee's analysis of Australian women's discursive shifts from a 'natural' to a 'normal' vulva [20]. Labiaplasty was constructed not only as a viable, but as an empowering, method to achieve this ideal:

some of you people are saying that only porn-stars get this procedure done and that girls shouldn't care if they are bigger. But having the problem where these girls are larger down there can be extremely ... embarrassing and why wouldn't someone do it to make them feel better about themselves. There is nothing wrong with getting this procedure and it is VERY common. GET it if you want it! You will feel much better and way more confident and that is good thing.

(L; I want labiaplasty; Yahoo UK #4)

I have recently undergone labiaplasty and straight away felt instant relief and my self-confidence is through the roof. ... You will not regret it, and as silly as it sounds it will change your lif. It has mine.

(C; I want labiaplasty; Yahoo UK #4)

In line with neoliberal self-improvement mandates, labiaplasty was constructed as a way to increase self-confidence – even, dramatically, to *change your life*. In this way, public discourse on forums echoes the empowering-psychologising discourse deployed by surgeons and the media [16, 17], constructing FGCS as a tool through which psychology operates.

Our analysis identified two ways a vulval ideal was evident: through a normalisation of a neat 'vulva' – this as the 'norm' is *conceptual*; it does not map onto material, fleshy reality, where vulval appearance is diverse [33] – and through the construction of 'protruding' labial tissue as both 'excessive' and 'freakish'. Larger labia minora, sometimes simply *visible* labia minora, were referred to using negative constructions such as 'worn-out', 'old-looking', 'overused', 'masculine', 'unattractive', 'disgusting' and 'sexually unappealing': "it

looked like a watermelon which had been hit with an axe" (U; I hate my vagina; Yahoo UK #2). Men's voices appeared as reported truths, or actual commentary, to validate the desirability of 'neatness': "I'm currently dating the love of my life, and I was so terribly devastated to discover that she doesn't have a neat little box ... it's SUCH a turn off for me" (J; I hate my vagina; Google UK #3).

Throughout the online discussions, a small and 'neat' vulva was held to represent femininity, youthfulness and desirability. And with the appearance, marketing and increased popularisation, and thus normalisation, of labiaplasty (discussed further later), it was (potentially) achievable even if your vulva did not meet the standard. It was indeed a *logical* course of action:

"I'm fourteen and I hate my vagina because of my big lips ... . It doesn't hurt me & is rarely uncomfortable. It just makes my self-esteem really low. I think I'm going to start saving up for this surgery now, so when I'm 18 I can get it done" (I; I want labiaplasty; Yahoo UK, #4).

For many, recounted embodied affect was deep and thorough, usually centred on disgust: "they disgust me, when I look in the mirror I just see ugliness ... " (C; I hate my vagina; Yahoo USA #3). Disgust is a powerful emotion, and one not unfamiliar to the experience of embodied womanhood [34, 35]. Some described the extreme lengths to which they had gone to resolve their labial concerns:

"I absolutely LOATHE mine ... my husband and I have even tried to burn them off with dry ice to see if that would work" (K; I hate my vagina; Google USA #5); "A few years ago I took my dad's carving knife and tried to slice it off" (B; I want labiaplasty; Yahoo UK #1).

The second patterned meaning "we can't all be Barbie" captured resistance to an idealised (small, neat, contained) vulval norm, constructing 'perfection' as non-existent and positioning the appropriate response as psychological reframing – 'learning to love yourself' – rather than surgical intervention. A diverse vulval *reality* was often contrasted with a (false) ideal or idea of normal, created by pornography:

Odds are you've watched porn so you've seen the "ideal" vagina. Pay no mind to that. Every vagina is as different as a thumb print. Just realize that EVERY girl is different down there and men don't usually dislike a single one.

(A; I hate my vagina; Yahoo USA #6)

> Stop watching porn. It's skewing your view of reality.
> *(M; are my labia normal? Yahoo NZ #4)*

Genital diversity was named, and desirability of *all* genital formations stated by some: "all are different, and all are beautiful" (T; are my labia normal? Google UK #3). Some evoked an individualising 'personal preference' discourse, but flipped what was valued: "small labia are just 'eh' to me. Gorgeous, sexy long labia are beautiful" (T; I hate my vagina; Yahoo UK #2). Lack of (sexuality) education, or *miseducation* in reference to pornography, was often situated as the problem [32], and information as the answer, which could have powerful impacts. For instance, in response to a *Hungry Beast* story about censorship of labia minora in media [36], R commented:

> Hungry Beast I actually love you so so so much. This has changed my life. For 10 years I have been convinced that I was a freak. I have never ever seen any vagina which actually looked like mine.
> *(R; I want labiaplasty; Yahoo NZ #5)*

> I am crying tears of relief right now.
> *(S, are my labia normal? Google UK #3)*

For R and S, information was revelatory, constructed as transformative to their selves. The data contained a sense of camaraderie, in a collectivised (lack of) understanding and knowledge – bearing contemporary echoes of the value of 'consciousness raising', a core activity for women's health movements [37]. Other accounts, however, highlighted that gaining information did not necessarily provide an easy solution:

> My inner labia are long and disgusting … Show me one fl'ing diagram of a vagina, like the ones in the doctor's office, that have big inner labia? Even professional models of vaginas are telling me that mine is weird and abnormal. But I am supposed to "love my body" right? It is impossible.
> *(A; I hate my vagina; Yahoo UK #2)*

This 'love your body' idea, that A challenges, was evident in various ways, articulating a neoliberal self-improving subject through a different mode, through claims that changing psychology was preferential to surgery:

> Guys post on this site every day saying they don't care and long is fine or even better than the shorter ones. Anyway you just need to learn to love your body … If it's really interfering with your life then you can get surgery but you could risk losing sensation down there, or becoming a person who needs surgery to "fix" every little problem with your body, and after this you would just obsess about something else.
> *(H; I hate my labia; Yahoo UK #9)*

Here, the *correct* response is to love your body – a surgical decision is 'allowed', but is pathologised at the same time. To shift from disgust to love is a potentially big ask. Recent critiques of the 'body positivity' movement [38] are relevant here. Some kind of 'neutrality' is perhaps not only a more realistic goal, but a mandate to 'love' can be part of unrealistic neoliberal and healthist perpetual body optimisation discourse, co-opted by, and perpetuated through, 'empowerment advertising' to women that penetrates deep into women's psyches [39]. This discourse is one that surgeon advertising directly evokes and reinforces, with claims of empowerment, amazing sex and psychological transformation [16, 17].

Threaded throughout the dataset were the voices of real (or claiming to be real) men, as well as reference to men as a general category. Men's voices expressed certain aesthetic preferences; claims of 'what men like/dislike' (see also [21, 40, 41]) appeared in various guises, positioned within a heteronormative framing as a relevant consideration. Men's voices provided reassurance that smaller isn't 'better'; men's voices expressed preference for 'the Barbie' vulva. In Alex Li's and my analysis of pubic hair practice, sexual partner preference was a key theme influencing women's pubic hair practice [26]. Often, a partner's preference was assumed or imagined – echoing the idea of 'the male in the head' explicated in Holland and colleagues' analysis of British youths' (hetero)sexual encounters [42]. The use of men's voices is troubling in two ways. First, men's tastes are often somehow treated as unchangeable, even *if* they are recognised as socio-culturally influenced (for instance, by pornography – an influence that has been questioned by some [43]). Second, it positions men as final arbiters of genital appearance. Combined, this gives more validity to what men might think than to what women might think about vulval appearance. It constructs a position of hetero-relational embodied aesthetics, but in a way in which power is not equally shared.

Selling the Vulva

How people make sense of vulval appearance does not occur outside of socio-cultural influence; nor do the options they perceive as available to them and/or desire to engage with [44]. Much of the early public narrative around genital cosmetic procedures came from surgeons [16], speaking into a context (noted earlier) of pre-existing strong negative vulval associations. I analysed the websites of a selection of surgeons from English-speaking countries who were offering FGCS [17]. I had systematically compiled a dataset of information from 20 websites (10 from US surgeons; 10 from UK, Australia, Canada and New Zealand surgeons) in 2005, a time when the surgery was still framed as fairly new and outside the typical offerings of gynaecologists or plastic surgeons. I focused on the way 'right' and 'wrong' genitalia were demarcated on the sites discursively, through the language used and visually, through before-and-after photos (see also [7]). The premise of my analysis is that reality is constructed [45], so language matters. Larger/visible labia minora were regularly discussed with language which suggested at best, redundancy, and at worst, pathology. The opposite – a vulva that is 'small' or 'neat', a vagina that is 'tight' – was explicitly and implicitly positioned as ideal. Through vague language, readers could exist in a state of comparative aesthetic uncertainty. Imagery worked alongside such uncertainty, to tell a transformational tale, and reveal a 'right' state. One small experimental study has suggested exposure to modified genital imagery can influence perceptions of normality and desirability [46].

I argued that the "sites work in multiple ways to sell both vulval distress and transformation. Certain morphologies are pathologized, implicitly and explicitly; certain morphologies are valorized. Women are invited into a medicalized regime of self-assessment and intervention to achieve the perfect vulva" ([17], p. 133). Psychology and affect were a key mode through which FGCS was legitimised, and promoted, on these sites. The genitalia were positioned as having the capacity to produce great psychological and emotional distress; the surgery, to resolve it. It offered a physical *and* psychological transformation, resulting in an empowered, bodily and sexually confident, sexually fulfilled woman. Of course the claims were not, necessarily, always *explicitly* stated in these terms. The material on surgeons' websites is increasingly recognised as partial and problematic [47]. A systematic review around impacts of online information identified similar themes, but highlighted a need for more research into the impact of the internet on the promotion and normalisation of these procedures [48]; others have urged caution in the public language around these procedures [49].

What Has Changed, and Why Should We Be Worried?

When I conducted that analysis, labiaplasty and related procedures could still be characterised as not-yet-normative, although situated within a trajectory of growth. Now, labiaplasty is everywhere: offered by many doctors as one of a plethora of genital interventions, as well as part of a complex cosmetic tourism industry that sees people travel to 'exotic' locations in search of cheaper procedures combined with some kind of 'holiday' [50]. Virtually daily, I receive Google alerts for 'labiaplasty' or 'designer vagina', mostly media stories or surgeon press releases. Genital procedures are now ubiquitous, but paradoxically they are still newsworthy; they are also still being questioned. I finish this chapter by briefly reflecting on the contemporary context (in the Global North), discussing mainstreaming and legitimisation, ongoing critique and the construction of the vulva as contemporary (economic) commodity.

Labiaplasty and other genital cosmetic procedures for the vulva/vagina have become (somewhat) mainstreamed and legitimised. This has occurred despite critique of both cultural hypocrisy and legal dubious standing when genital 'cosmetic' procedures are considered alongside laws banning 'female genital mutilation' (e.g., [51]). By mainstreaming, I am referring to a shift in socio-cultural positioning – from something fringe or extreme, something shocking, to something more 'everyday', more mundane, more 'normal'. Although extensive media stories in one way construct labiaplasty and their ilk *as newsworthy* and by definition unusual, the constant presence of the topic *normalises* the idea through keeping it in everyday discourse, normalises genital modification as something that people do. And stories which tell of (massive) increases in numbers having labiaplasty (etc.), or expressing interest [52–54], similarly work to make such procedures a 'happening thing' – even if they contain content that is (also) critical of it.

A mainstreaming also occurs as more and more surgeons offer labiaplasty and other genital procedures through private practice (as well as within public health systems). Google labiaplasty, and if you live in a city in the Anglo-West, you will probably find a clinic near you. It appears to have become a necessary procedure to offer, like rhinoplasty or breast enlargement. Various studies continue to (claim to) demonstrate 'positive outcomes' (e.g.,

[55]) and point to the procedure as 'safe' and carrying 'a high satisfaction rate' [56, 57]. This does not mean it *will* be successful – there is now an industry in labiaplasty repair [58], sometimes with the same surgeons who pioneered labiaplasty [59] – but it adds to visibility and therefore normalises. Surgeons continue to publish around their techniques (e.g., [60]), and the establishment of a professional body in 2004 – the International Society of Cosmetogynecology [61] – does *legitimising* work, aligned to mainstreaming, as well as offering training and promotional activities. From the *outside*, labiaplasty now appears as a normalised and legitimate form of cosmetic alteration. But it remains contested, within, as well as outside, the medical profession [62]. The UK's Nuffield Council on Bioethics, in their major 2017 report on the ethics of cosmetic procedures [63], highlighted many concerns related to FGCS (see also [64]), and noted the way dissatisfaction with body parts is promoted throughout the entire cosmetic surgery industry.

Professional critique has continued – from initial cautions issued in a 2007 opinion statement by the American College of Obstetricians and Gynecologists (ACOG) [65] and the corresponding Australasian body in 2008 [66]. For instance, the Society of Obstetricians and Gynaecologists of Canada (SOGC) evaluated evidence in 2013 and concluded that

> The weight of evidence currently available does not support female genital cosmetic surgery, and the proliferation of non-medically indicated surgery to the genital area is of great concern. ... The SOGC's position does not support non-medically indicated female genital cosmetic surgery procedures considering the available evidence of efficacy and safety. ([67], p. 1112)

They also specifically addressed the case of adolescent patients, evidencing a growing 'demand' among younger populations and adolescents seeking medical advice on perceived labial abnormality [68]. ACOG very recently produced guidelines *specifically* addressing labial (and breast) surgery in adolescents, reiterating, "although there may be a perception that labiaplasty is a minor procedure, serious complications can occur" ([69], p. 18).

Concerns about the rise of labiaplasty, understood as often based in a 'lack of knowledge' of genital diversity, have promoted the appearance of various sites – usually online [70, 71], but sometimes in book

[72] or art form (e.g., British artist Jamie McCartney's paster-cast artwork "Great Wall of Vagina" [73]) – aimed at demonstrating vulval diversity, and hence normalising it. Such resources *may* have some impact on knowledge [74], or shame [75], and are hence a vital part of disrupting the idea that labial visibility is unusual, weird or wrong [31]. The inadequacy of genital information in medical-training texts has been noted [76]. But bodily desires, psychology and practices are more complex than just about *information*. We are *all* socio-culturally located, including doctors [77], and extrication from implicit, embedded norms is complex. And although we do not yet have complex analysis of women who get labiaplasty, there is some indication that their genital distress is more impactful on their lives than on those of women not seeking labial surgery [78], even if their genitalia are 'normal' [79].

Finally, I want to highlight some intensifications that have occurred really within the last decade, which suggest the vulvo-vaginal region can now firmly be located as *commodity*. Coincidental with the shame and taboos that *have been* strongly associated with these genitalia [18, 80], *public* narratives around genital appearance and genital change are commonplace. Furthermore, a veritable industry of products and services has developed, both those which reinforce narrow (aesthetic) norms, shame and disgust, and those which are resistant. Regardless of *what specific aspect* of vulvo-vaginal care or practice is being sold, all construct the vulva/vagina *as commodity*. In a quite fundamental way, the vulva/vagina become conceptualised as distinct bodily parts that can be – or may be *required* to be – targets for our (aesthetic) intervention. I conceptualise this as a self-reinforcing system: once the vulva/vagina has been constructed as a site of attention/intervention, it makes (capitalist) sense to develop products and services; as more and more of these appear, the idea of vulva/vagina as commodity and site for attention/intervention is reinforced. (For a fascinating and relevant analysis of these changes within a biopolitics framework, whereby an appropriate and *useful* vulva/vagina is now required, see [81].)

Something I had not anticipated was the appearance of an intense 'well-being' movement, meshed in with capitalism. In retrospect, it is obvious it would happen. We have a perfect storm of a socio-cultural history of shame and distress, and a gendered neoliberal self-perfecting subject aligned with healthist imperatives to be the best you can be – both overall, and in specific ways. Scrutinisation of women's bodies, sexualities, selves has extensified and intensified, from macro to micro surveillance. In this context, various highly critiqued products are being developed, promoted and sold, from vaginal steaming [82] to a powder made from oak galls to tighten the vagina [83].

It is easy to dismiss such products as ridiculous fads – and indeed, we ought to question and challenge their validity (84). But there seems to be continued media appetite for the latest 'scandalous' story of what women are *now* doing with their genitalia – such as the woman who turned her post-labiaplasty excised tissue into a pendant [85]. But such stories (and products) rely on, and reinforce, the dual narrative that the vulva/vagina is never quite right, and *should* be improved; that vulvar aesthetics *matter* [86].[3] And through this, it has become commodified. While we might be tempted to mock these products, and sometimes the people who seek them out, our analysis needs compassion. It also needs to come back to an historically oriented gendered-power analysis, in which we recognise that genito-reproductive medicine has not served 'women's' interests well – from the experimentation on black women's bodies through which 'modern' gynaecology was founded, a subject of recent public discussion [87], to the current vaginal mesh scandal [88]. And neither has society.

The New Normal

Cosmetic *surgeries* are among the most common of the plethora of genital procedures aimed at vulval/vaginal aesthetics (and function) that have appeared in the last few decades. Surgeons (in private practice) doing 'FGCS' are not in the simple business of responding to a problem. Although risk and vulnerability are important, a focus on these elides other factors. Not just in the business of selling the 'perfect' vulva, such surgeons are also implicitly involved in constructing or legitimising problems and (re)constructing norms. They are reorienting our sociocultural frameworks for thinking about what a vulva *should* look like it, and indeed what having one means, in terms of embodied obligations and opportunities. They are in the business of selling the *normal* vulva. But the normal vulva is no longer the 'natural' vulva – it is a modifiable, and visually modified, vulva, one

that requires attention and work, sometimes at great cost and with great risk, and which usually precludes visible labia minora.

References

1. Scott E. A surgeon says women are getting designer vagina surgery to look better in leggings. *Metrocouk*. 6 October 2017. Available from: http://metro.co.uk/2017/10/06/a-surgeon-says-women-are-getting-designer-vagina-surgery-to-look-better-in-leggings-6981111/

2. Braun V. *Rethinking Ruskin's wife's vulva*. In Elias AS, Gill R, Scharff C (eds), *Aesthetic labour: Rethinking beauty politics in neoliberalism*. Basingstoke: Palgrave; 2017, pp. 67–82.

3. Crann SE, Jenkins A, Money DM, O'Doherty KC. Women's genital body work: Health, hygiene and beauty practices in the production of idealized female genitalia. *Feminism Psychol*. 2017:0959353517711964.

4. Braun V. Female genital cutting around the globe: A matter of reproductive justice? In Chrisler JC (ed), *Reproductive justice: A global concern*. Santa Barbara, CA: Praeger; 2012, pp. 29–55.

5. Green FJ. From clitoridectomies to 'designer vaginas': The medical construction of heteronormative female bodies and sexuality through female genital cutting. *Sex Evol Gender*. 2005;7(2):153–87.

6. McDougall LJ. Towards a clean slit: How medicine and notions of normality are shaping female genital aesthetics. *Cult Health Sex*. 2013;15(7):774–87.

7. Moran C, Lee C. Selling genital cosmetic surgery to healthy women: A multimodal discourse analysis of Australian surgical websites. *Crit Discourse Stud*. 2013;10(4):373–91.

8. Tiefer L. Female genital cosmetic surgery: Freakish or inevitable? Analysis from medical marketing, bioethics, and feminist theory. *Feminism Psychol*. 2008;18(4):466–79.

9. Triffin M. WARNING: These doctors may be dangerous to your vagina. *Cosmopolitan*. 2010 July; 159–61.

10. Tiefer L. Activism on the medicalization of sex and female genital cosmetic surgery by the New View Campaign in the United States. *Reprod Health Matters*. 2010;18(35):56–63.

11. Braun V. "The women are doing it for themselves": The rhetoric of choice and agency around female genital 'cosmetic surgery'. *Aust Feminist Stud*. 2009;24 (60):233–49.

12. Braun V. Female genital cosmetic surgery: A critical review of current knowledge and contemporary debates. *J Womens Health*. 2010;19(7). Available from: http://doi.org/10.1089/jwh.2009.1728

---

[3] A recent surgeon-authored article, for instance, promoted the concept of "genital beautification" [88].

13. Braun V. Female genital cutting. In Teo T (ed), *Encyclopedia of critical psychology*. New York: Springer; 2014, pp. 693–7.

14. Braun V. Female genital cosmetic surgery. In Whelehan P, Bolin A (eds), *International encyclopedia of human sexuality*, Vol. I. Malden, MA: Wiley-Blackwell; 2015, pp. 372–4.

15. Braun V, Tiefer L. The 'designer vagina' and the pathologisation of female genital diversity: Interventions for change. *Radical Psychol.* 2010;18(1): [online]. Available from: www.radicalpsychology.org/vol8-1/brauntiefer.html

16. Braun V. In search of (better) sexual pleasure: Female genital 'cosmetic' surgery. *Sexualities.* 2005;8(4):407–24.

17. Braun V. Selling the 'perfect' vulva. In Heyes C, Jones M (eds), *Cosmetic surgery: A feminist primer.* Farnham, UK: Ashgate; 2009, pp. 133–49.

18. Braun V, Wilkinson S. Liability or asset? Women talk about the vagina. *Psychol Women Sect Rev.* 2003;5(2):28–42.

19. Fahs B. Genital panics: Constructing the vagina in women's qualitative narratives about pubic hair, menstrual sex, and vaginal self-image. *Body Image.* 2014;11(3):210–8.

20. Moran C, Lee C. 'Everyone wants a vagina that looks less like a vagina': Australian women's views on dissatisfaction with genital appearance. *J Health Psychol.* 2016:1359105316637588.

21. Mullinax M, Herbenick D, Schick V, Sanders SA, Reece M. In their own words: A qualitative content analysis of women's and men's preferences for women's genitals. *Sex Educ.* 2015;15(4):421–36.

22. Herbenick D, Schick V, Reece M, Sanders S, Dodge B, Fortenberry JD. The Female Genital Self-Image Scale (FGSIS): Results from a nationally representative probability sample of women in the United States. *J Sex Med.* 2011;8(1):158–66.

23. Fashemi B, Delaney ML, Onderdonk AB, Fichorova RN. Effects of feminine hygiene products on the vaginal mucosal biome. *Microb Ecol Health Dis.* 2013;24(1):19703.

24. Jenkins AL, Crann SE, Money DM, O'Doherty KC. "Clean and fresh": Understanding women's use of vaginal hygiene products. *Sex Roles.* 2018;78(9–10): 697–709.

25. Braun V, Kitzinger C. 'Snatch', 'hole', or 'honey pot'? Semantic categories and the problem of non-specificity in female genital slang. *J Sex Res.* 2001;38:146–58.

26. Li AY, Braun V. Pubic hair and its removal: A practice beyond the personal. *Feminism Psychol.* 2017;27(3): 336–56.

27. Elias A, Gill R, Scharff C. Aesthetic labour: Beauty politics in neoliberalism. In Elias AS, Gill R, Scharff C (eds), *Aesthetic labour: Rethinking beauty politics in neoliberalism.* London: Palgrave Macmillan; 2017, pp. 3–49.

28. Giles D. Online discussion. Forums. In Braun V, Clarke V, Gray D (eds), *Collecting qualitative data: A practical guide to textual, media and virtual techniques.* Cambridge: Cambridge University Press; 2017, pp. 166–88.

29. Hookway N. Archives of everyday life. In Braun V, Clarke V, Gray D (eds), *Collecting qualitative data: A practical guide to textual, media and virtual techniques.* Cambridge: Cambridge University Press; 2017, pp. 144–65.

30. Braun V, Clarke V. Using thematic analysis in psychology. *Qual Res Psychol.* 2006;3(2):77–101.

31. Howarth C, Hayes J, Simonis M, Temple-Smith M. 'Everything's neatly tucked away': Young women's views on desirable vulval anatomy. *Cult Health Sex.* 2016:1–16.

32. Howarth H, Sommer V, Jordan FM. Visual depictions of female genitalia differ depending on source. *J Med Humanit.* 2010;36(2):75–9.

33. Lloyd J, Crouch NS, Minto CL, Liao L-M, Creighton SM. Female genital appearance: 'Normality' unfolds. *Br J Obstet Gynaecol.* 2005;112:643–6.

34. Chrisler JC. Leaks, lumps, and lines: Stigma and women's bodies. *Psychol Women Q.* 2011;35(2): 202–14.

35. Fahs B. The dreaded body: Disgust and the production of "appropriate" femininity. *J Gender Stud.* 2017;26(2): 184–96.

36. Drysdale K. Healing it to a single crease. *Hungry Beast*: ABC Australia; 2010.

37. Turshen M. *Women's health movements: A global force for change.* New York: Palgrave Macmillan; 2007.

38. Meltzer M. Forget body positivity: How about body neutrality? *The Cut.* March 1, 2017. Available from: www.thecut.com/2017/03/forget-body-positivity-how-about-body-neutrality.html

39. Gill R, Elias AS. 'Awaken your incredible': Love your body discourses and postfeminist contradictions. *Int J Media Cult Polit.* 2014;10(2):179–88.

40. Horrocks E, Iyer J, Askern A, Becuzzi N, Vangaveti V, Rane A. Individual male perception of female genitalia. *Int Urogynecol J.* 2016;27(2):307–13.

41. Mazloomdoost D, Crisp CC, Westermann LB, et al. Survey of male perceptions regarding the vulva. *Am J Obstet Gynecol.* 2015;213(5):731.e1–731.e9.

42. Holland J, Ramazanoglu C, Sharpe S, Thomson R. *The male in the head: Young people, heterosexuality and power*. London: The Tufnell Press; 1998.

43. Jones B, Nurka C. Labiaplasty and pornography: A preliminary investigation. *Porn Stud*. 2015;2 (1):62–75.

44. Sharp G, Tiggemann M, Mattiske J. Predictors of consideration of labiaplasty: An extension of the tripartite influence model of beauty ideals. *Psychol Women Q*. 2015;39(2):182–93.

45. Burr V. *Social constructionism*. 2nd ed. London: Psychology Press; 2003.

46. Moran C, Lee C. What's normal? Influencing women's perceptions of normal genitalia: An experiment involving exposure to modified and nonmodified images. *BJOG*. 2014;121(6):761–6.

47. Liao L-M, Taghinejadi N, Creighton SM. An analysis of the content and clinical implications of online advertisements for female genital cosmetic surgery. *BMJ Open*. 2012;2(6):e001908.

48. Mowat H, McDonald K, Dobson AS, Fisher J, Kirkman M. The contribution of online content to the promotion and normalisation of female genital cosmetic surgery: A systematic review of the literature. *BMC Womens Health*. 2015;15(1):1–10.

49. Ashong AC, Batta HE. Sensationalising the female pudenda: An examination of public communication of aesthetic genital surgery. *Global J Health Sci*. 2012;5(2): 153–65.

50. Holliday R, Bell D, Jones M, Hardy K, Hunter E, Probyn E, et al. Beautiful face, beautiful place: Relational geographies and gender in cosmetic surgery tourism websites. *Gender Place Cult*. 2015;22 (1):90–106.

51. Avalos L. Female genital mutilation and designer vaginas in Britain: Crafting an effective legal and policy framework. *Vanderbilt JTransnatl Law*. 2015;48:621–706.

52. Forster K. Labiaplasty: Vaginal surgery 'world's fastest-growing cosmetic procedure', say plastic surgeons. *Independent*. 12 July 2017. Available from: www .independent.co.uk/news/health/labiaplasty-vagina-su rgery-cosmetic-procedure-plastic-study-interna tional-society-aesthetic-plastic-a7837181.html

53. Holloway K. The labiaplasty boom: Why are women desperate for the perfect vagina? *Alternet*. 13 February 2015. Available from: www.alternet.org/news-amp-po litics/labiaplasty-boom-why-are-women-desperate-perfect-vagina

54. Sullivan R. New survey finds more women want female genital cosmetic surgery. *Newscomau*. 5 May 2016. Available from: www.news.com.au/lifestyle/beauty/co smetic-surgery/new-survey-finds-more-women-want-

female-genital-cosmetic-surgery/news-story/ 1e45b24b22a7676ddbcf0a44447a3554

55. Veale D, Naismith I, Eshkevari E, et al. Psychosexual outcome after labiaplasty: A prospective case-comparison study. *Int Urogynecol J*. 2014;25(6): 831–9.

56. Motakef S, Rodriguez-Feliz J, Chung MT, Ingargiola MJ, Wong VW, Patel A. Vaginal labiaplasty: Current practices and a simplified classification system for labial protrusion. *Plast Reconstr Surg*. 2015;135(3): 774–88.

57. Goodman MP. Female genital cosmetic and plastic surgery: A review. *J Sex Med*. 2011;8(6):1813–25.

58. Alter G. Botched labiaplasty revision surgery: About the procedure 2017. Available from: www .labiaplastyrevisionsurgeon.com/botched-labiaplasty/

59. Alter GJ. A new technique for aesthetic labia minora reduction. *Ann Plast Surg*. 1998;40(3):287–90.

60. Abbed T, Mussat F, Cohen M. Origami model for central wedge labiaplasty: A simple educational model with video tutorial. *Aesthet Surg J*. 2017;37(10):NP132-NP6.

61. International Society of Cosmetogynecology. 2014. Available from: www.iscgyn.com/en/aboutus

62. Barbara G, Facchin F, Meschia M, Vercellini P. "The first cut is the deepest": A psychological, sexological and gynecological perspective on female genital cosmetic surgery. *Acta Obstet Gynecol Scand*. 2015;94(9):915–20.

63. Bioethics. NCo. Cosmetic procedures: Ethical issues. 2017.

64. Edmonds A. Can medicine be aesthetic? *Med Anthropol Q*. 2013;27(2):233–52.

65. Committee on Gynecologic Practice, American College of Obstetricians and Gynecologists. ACOG Committee Opinion No. 378: Vaginal "rejuvenation" and cosmetic vaginal procedures. *Obstet Gynecol*. 2007;110(3):737–8.

66. The Royal Australian and New Zealand College of Obstetricians and Gynaecologists. Vaginal 'rejuvenation' and cosmetic vaginal procedures. New College Statement C-Gyn 24. Melbourne: The Royal Australian and New Zealand College of Obstetricians and Gynaecologists; 2008.

67. Shaw D, Lefebvre G, Bouchard C, et al. Female genital cosmetic surgery. *J Obstet Gynaecol Can*. 2013;35(12): 1108–12.

68. Michala L, Koliantzaki S, Antsaklis A. Protruding labia minora: Abnormal or just uncool? *J Psychosom Obstet Gynecol*. 2011;32(3):154–6.

69. Committee on Gynecologic Practice, American College of Obstetricians and Gynecologists. ACOG

Committee Opinion No. 668: Breast and labial surgery in adolescents. *Obstet Gynecol.* 2017;129:e17–9.

70. The Labia Library 2011. www.labialibrary.org.au/

71. The Vulva Gallery 2017. www.thevulvagallery.com/

72. Karras N. *Petals.* San Diego, CA: Crystal River Publishing; 2003.

73. McCartney J. Great Wall of Vagina. Fine Art Studios. Available from: www.greatwallofvagina.co.uk/home

74. Sharp G, Tiggemann M. Educating women about normal female genital appearance variation. *Body Image.* 2016;16:70–8.

75. Frischherz M. Affective agency and transformative shame: The voices behind the great wall of vagina. *Womens Stud Commun.* 2015;38(3):251–72.

76. Andrikopoulou M, Michala L, Creighton S, Liao L. The normal vulva in medical textbooks. *J Obstet Gynaecol.* 2013;33(7):648–50.

77. Reitsma W, Mourits MJ, Koning M, Pascal A, van der Lei B. No (wo) man is an island—the influence of physicians' personal predisposition to labia minora appearance on their clinical decision making: A cross-sectional survey. *J Sex Med.* 2011;8(8):2377–85.

78. Veale D, Eshkevari E, Ellison N, et al. Psychological characteristics and motivation of women seeking labiaplasty. *Psychol Med.* 2014;44(3):555–66.

79. Crouch NS, Deans R, Michala L, Liao LM, Creighton SM. Clinical characteristics of well women seeking labial reduction surgery: A prospective study. *BJOG.* 2011;118(12):1507–10.

80. Braun V, Wilkinson S. Socio-cultural representations of the vagina. *J Reprod Infant Psychol.* 2001;19:17–32.

81. Rodrigues S. From vaginal exception to exceptional vagina: The biopolitics of female genital cosmetic surgery. *Sexualities.* 2012;15(7):778–94.

82. Vandenburg T, Braun V. 'Basically, it's sorcery for your vagina': Unpacking Western representations of vaginal steaming. *Cult Health Sex.* 2017;19(4): 470–85.

83. Oak Gall for Vaginal Tightening and Rejuvenation FEMALE RENEWAL SOLUTION; 2017. Available from: http://intivar.greenliveforever.com/oak_gall_va ginal_tightening.html

84. Weiss S. Health. 17 August 2017. Available from: www .self.com/story/vaginal-products-and-treatments

85. Woman turns discarded vagina skin into jewelry. *The Province.* 1 October 2017. Available from: http:// theprovince.com/news/world/woman-turns-discar ded-vagina-skin-into-jewelry

86. Cihantimur B, Herold C. Genital beautification: A concept that offers more than reduction of the labia minora. *Aesth Plast Surg.* 2013;37(6):1128–33.

87. Spettel S, White MD. The portrayal of J. Marion Sims' controversial surgical legacy. *J Urol.* 2011;185(6): 2424–7.

88. Peck T. Labour calls for public inquiry into vaginal mesh implants. *Independent.* 17 October 2017. Available from: www.independent.co.uk/news/uk/poli tics/vaginal-mesh-implants-surgical-mesh-labour-pub lic-inquiry-sharon-hodgson-a8005786.html

The History of Female Genital Cosmetic Surgery in the United States

From Marginal to Mainstream

Sarah B. Rodriguez

"Is female genital cosmetic surgery going mainstream?" So queried the headline of a June 2017 article in *Ob. Gyn. News* reporting on a debate at the American College of Obstetricians and Gynecologists' (ACOG) annual clinical meeting the preceding month [1]. The question of whether these surgeries were becoming mainstream was based in part on a report that physicians performed 12,666 labiaplasties in 2016 in the United States, an increase of 39% from 2015, according to the American Society of Plastic Surgeons (ASPS) [2]. These findings supported the contention made by those in plastic surgery that female genital cosmetic surgery (FGCS) was becoming more widespread in cosmetic surgery and gynecology [3]. What was driving this growth? According to Iglesia, a physician who engaged in the debate, it was the "highly-curated, and extensively retouched, images on social media and the mainstream media" that were "leaving women and men with little idea of the real range of normal female external genitalia" [4].

Implicit in the foregoing question is that FGCS had once been uncommon. Assuming that FGCS – surgeries that include the removal of parts of the labia, clitoral unhooding, and vaginal tightening – are "going mainstream," how did surgeries that were once considered uncommon rise to the point of possibly becoming standard within cosmetic surgery and gynecology? As FGCS is not a single surgery, and the number of FGCS procedures and their historical precedents would have led to an unwieldy chapter, I focus on labiaplasty, the most commonly performed FGCS [5]. To examine my question – how did these once uncommon surgeries rise to become mainstream surgical offerings – I examine how physicians discussed labiaplasty in their published articles. Specifically, I consider two changes between 1971 and 2008: first, a change in the way physicians discussed the diversity of labial appearance and second, a change from

physicians regarding enlarged labia as an uncommon condition, and labiaplasty rarely indicated, to referring to labiaplasty as an increasingly popular procedure requested by women. I then contextualize these changes within larger changes in medical practice.

Before I begin, a few notes on the limits of this history. First, as I examine the history of labiaplasty only as an elective, cosmetic procedure, I do not consider reconstructive surgeries for diseases such as cancer, or the reduction of labias defined as hypertrophied performed on individuals deemed to have congenital conditions of sex ambiguity. Nor does this chapter consider transsexual surgical reassignment procedures, or practices that usually fall under the nomenclature of female genital mutilation/female genital cutting, though others – both those critiquing as well as practicing FGCS – have drawn connections and distinctions between them [6, 7]. And I do not examine labiaplasty techniques, or the debate within gynecology about whether gynecologists should perform FGCS [8, 9]. Finally, though I discuss the use of labiaplasty by clinicians outside the United States, I more narrowly focus on changes to medical practice in the United States.

From Reassurance of Diversity to the Patient's Perspective

The first published article on labiaplasty appeared in 1971, and between 1971 and 2008, 20 reports on labiaplasty appeared in medical journals [8]. Beginning with the first article discussing labiaplasty, clinicians noted female patients came to them out of concern about the size of their labia. In his 1971 article, American gynecologist Capraro wrote about occasions when practitioners would see girls "with marked hypertrophy of the labia minora" and the girl – or her mother – would be worried about it as an "abnormality" [10]. French gynecologist Rouzier and colleagues in 2000 similarly noted "large labia projecting beyond the labia majora are occasionally a concern among adolescent and adult women" [11].

However, some clinicians noted that when presented with a patient concerned about the size or shape of her labia, they found reassuring the patient about the diversity of female genitalia usually sufficed. Capraro said patients usually only needed "reassurance that this is simply a variant of normal, such as big ears or big feet" [10]. In 1988, American gynecologists Gowen and Martin wrote "often all that is needed" was to reassure the woman variation was normal [12]. In 1989, American physicians Chavis, LaFerla, and Niccolini wrote "in many cases concern about vulvar appearance can be resolved by reassurance alone" [13]. Similarly, in 1997, Australian physician Fliegner noted women concerned with "labia minora projecting beyond the labia majora" often "require reassurance only" [14]. In a 1999 article, Netherland physicians Maas and Hage agreed, writing "concerns about the appearance of labia minora extending beyond the labia majora can often be alleviated by explaining variation in size is normal" [15]. In 2004, Japanese gynecologists wrote that most patients who "subjectively reported hypertrophic labia minora require reassurance" of the diversity of female genitalia [16]. In 2008, New Zealand practitioners Lynch and colleagues wrote "females need to be reassured that hypertrophy of the labia minora is simply a variant of the normal" [17].

By around the time of publication of Lynch's article, however, clinicians writing about labiaplasty seemed to stop noting often all that was needed was reassuring the patient of genital diversity. Though some physicians continued to note that "normal female genitalia vary widely," they did not state whether this was something they told their patients [18]. Instead, some practitioners suggested enlarged labia were not part of the diversity of female vulvas. For example, in 2010, American gynecologists Reddy and Laufer wrote that once enlarged labia "was considered a variant of normal anatomy," suggesting this was no longer so [19]. Echoing this sentiment, Chinese physicians in 2012 wrote "[p]reviously, it was believed that hypertrophy of the labia minora is a variant of normal anatomy" [20]. Though Canadian physicians Lista and colleagues wrote in 2015 "it was important for plastic surgeons to stress that a patient demonstrate a variance of normal when this is the case," since the "essence of aesthetic surgery is that plastic surgeons operate on patients who have a normal appearance with the goal being to improve their appearance," noting to a patient genital diversity did not seem relevant to cosmetic surgery [21].

Diversity in genital appearance, then, changed from being clinically normal to normality at the discretion of the woman. This was because, as Colombian physicians wrote in 2012, women "can now compare themselves, see how others look, and decide if their genital appearance is acceptable or not" [18]. Clinicians supported the assertion that women could decide if their genitals needed surgery by stating there was "little consensus on the definition of labia minora hypertrophy" [22]. Possibly some of this shift – from reassurance about genital diversity to differing to the woman's view of genital (ab)normality – can be tied to changes in the doctor–patient relationship, with physicians being less patriarchal and more respectful of the autonomous decision-making of their patients, a change that began in the 1970s in the United States [23]. But this change also occurred during a time of additional changes in American medicine, something I address shortly.

From Uncommon Exceptions to an Increasingly Common Offering

Though physicians writing about labiaplasty from 1971 until around 2008 often noted they reassured their patients about genital diversity, starting with the 1971 article, clinicians also noted there were exceptions to reassurance. Capraro wrote if the condition was "embarrassing to the patient, or is a source of irritation, excision, and plastic repair, may be done" [10]. In 1976, American gynecologist Radman suggested that if "abnormalities" resulted in symptoms "that are incompatible with comfort and personal hygiene" then "corrective operative procedures" should be done [24]. Similarly, in 1978, two Canadian physicians discussed surgically reducing the size of the labia of two patients who presented with "floppy" labia resulting in chafing and discomfort [25]. And in 1984, Americans Hodgkinson and Hait wrote, "reduction of the labia minora may improve the physical comfort and sexuality of some women" [7].

Similarly, Chavis and colleagues argued that, in a case such as the one they reported – when the woman "experiences mechanical difficulties, such as dyspareunia, pressure under tight clothing and difficulty cleansing after elimination because of aberrant labia," – then "elongated labia may be amenable to effective and safe surgical treatment" [13]. Likewise, in 1995,

American gynecologists Laufer and Galvin wrote that while "hypertrophy of the labia minora" was a variant of "normal anatomy," "occasionally a patient will complain of severe symptoms that require intervention." The most common, they believed, were "poor hygiene and problems with sexual relations" as well as a "poor sense of self-esteem" [26]. Gowen and Martin wrote there were "women with legitimate complaints" making "surgical reduction acceptable and necessary." Such complaints included "pinching or chaffing when walking or sitting," hygiene issues related to menstruation or bowel movements, or "interference with vaginal penetration during intercourse," and for these patients "surgical reduction of the labia minora" is "not unreasonable" [12].

Fliegner agreed, writing that though he felt labiaplasty was "rarely required," if the labia were enlarged to a "gross degree," it warranted surgical reduction for "functional, aesthetic, or social reasons" [14]. Similarly, Maas and Hage noted enlarged labia minora "can be functionally or psychosocially bothersome," including problems with irritation, "personal hygiene during menses or after bowel movements, interference with sexual intercourse, and discomfort during cycling, walking, or sitting are generally accepted as indications for surgical reduction." Additionally, "aesthetic concerns influence the psychological and social well-being of the patient" and were further reasons for surgery [15]. Rouzier and colleagues noted while "hypertrophy of the labia minora is not a pathologic condition," when the "patient has aesthetic or functional concerns, labia minora reduction should be proposed" [11].

Note clinicians here were suggesting that in some cases labiaplasty was indicated, but for particular, uncommon indications. The few articles published from the 1970s through the 1990s and the small number of patients in the articles – until a 1999 article reported on 13 cases, no one reported on more than three cases – signifies concern for enlarged labia to the extent surgery was proposed was unusual. Some of the clinicians writing during this time explicitly noted the infrequency of the procedure. To illustrate, Chavis and colleagues noted women's external genitalia "represent an area on which plastic surgery is performed infrequently" [13]. In a particularly interesting, and unusual, instance, an editorial comment before Fliegner's article stated the journal "accepted this paper for publication since we agree with the author that it is rare for patients to request surgery for enlargement of the labia minora" [14]. Similarly, Rouzier and colleagues noted they wished to

"stress" that labiaplasty constituted a "very minor part of our practice" [11]. Sakamoto and colleagues wrote "medical intervention is usually unnecessary," while in 2005, Brazilian cosmetic surgeon Munhoz and colleagues wrote, "aesthetic surgery of the female genitalia is an uncommon procedure" [16, 27]. In 1998, Alter wrote, "aesthetic surgery of the female genitalia has not been of significant interest among physicians" [28].

However, in articles published in 1989 and 1995, the authors speculated on whether physicians should perhaps offer labiaplasty because conceivably more women and adolescent girls were concerned about the size of their labias. In 1995, Laufer and Galvin stated that with the "increasing emphasis in society on physical appearance, women are more concerned about their bodies and any perceived imperfections," a "trend" that could result in gynecologists seeing "more patients seeking treatment of asymptomatic labial enlargement" [26]. Similarly, in 1989, Chavis and colleagues wrote that as women were "socialized to consider their genitalia as 'off limits' for discussion," some women were perhaps reluctant to discuss concerns with their doctors about the appearance of their labia. These women "may be silently troubled," and the authors wondered if there could be "a considerable number of women" who were "not being helped as much as they could be because they are too uncomfortable to voice their concerns or because their physicians are reluctant to view the problem as one worthy of surgical treatment" [13]. Perhaps there was, these comments suggested, an unmet interest in labiaplasty; perhaps more women were concerned about the aesthetics of their labia or had issues concerning chaffing.

These speculations came to fruition a decade later, as physicians started noting a growing interest in the surgery. For example, Alter in 2008 wrote, "demand for labia minora reduction has increased" [29]. Additionally, in the cosmetic surgery newsletter article "The Shape of Things to Come," the author suggested labiaplasty be added to the "popular list" of surgeries, as it was "experiencing a growth spurt" [30]. Others noted the growth of labiaplasty was a result of the increased interest in the "aesthetics of female genitalia" as "an area of concern among women over the past 10 years" [31]. This increased interest, physicians asserted, rose from popular media images of female genitals.

Clinicians noted starting in the 1980s the role the media played in women's perceptions of their genitals. In 1984, Hodgkinson and Hait wrote the

35

"exposure of female genitals in popular magazines allows more critical appraisal of female genital aesthetics by both men and women" [7]. But in photographs of women appearing in either tight clothing or naked in women's magazines, a study in 2002 found the vulva area was typically obscured or depicted as smoothly curving between the woman's thighs [32]. These images, then, failed to show the diversity of the genitalia and instead showed genitalia as uniformly flat and smooth.

In addition, however, to women's magazines as a reference for labia depictions, clinicians also referenced sexually explicit media as influencing ideas. Alter in 1998 wrote "women have become more aware of differences in genital appearance owing to publication of nude pictures in magazines and nude presentation in movies" [28]. Labiaplasty practitioners when interviewed in the popular media often mentioned the influence of pornography as a driver of the surgery. For example, in a 2004 article, physician Matlock said, "I can't tell you how many pages and pages of pornographic material women have brought into me saying 'I want to look like this'" [33]. Young, the chair of the ASPS's emerging trends task force, said in 2005 he thought the rise of labiaplasty was a result of the "mainstreaming of pornography." Male partners "see images on the Internet or in movies and comment" to their female partners, resulting in the woman thinking "'I didn't know I was 'abnormal.' Or she doesn't think she's as cute," Young said [34]. Other clinicians also pointed to explicit media motivating women to seek labiaplasty to be more in line with models in *Playboy* [35].

An analysis of *Playboy* centerfolds from 2007 to 2008, however, found the exposed labia resembled that of a prepubescent female, giving a narrow view of female genitalia [36]. Regardless, then, of why physicians stopped noting they reassured women of normality and started instead implying normality was at the discretion of the woman, this change occurred in parallel to when clinicians also began noting women approached them with images of the labia that failed to show the diversity of the labia – indeed that portrayed a very narrow view. And it also occurred alongside an increase in the popular media covering labiaplasty.

Beginning in the mid to late 2000s, clinicians noted the media as driving an increased interest from women in labiaplasty. Alter, for example, in 2008 noted that the increase in demand for labiaplasty

was because of "recent media coverage of this operation" [29]. Many FGCS practitioners over the next decade similarly credited the rise in patients' demand for labiaplasty to the increase in lay press coverage [37]. Indeed, a report in *Ob. Gyn. News* in 2010 noted while there had only been "a handful of papers in scientific journals" regarding labiaplasty, this number was "dwarfed by coverage of the procedure in women's magazines and the lay press" [9].

Popular Media and the Increase of Labiaplasty

The first popular article regarding labiaplasty appeared in 1994. In the *For Women First* article "Intimate Surgery," reporter Meyer interviewed "Dawn," a 27-year-old woman embarrassed by what she considered her enlarged labia. Dawn felt "like a freak" and told Meyer she could not "wear certain outfits – nothing clingy or sexy." Dawn was considering labiaplasty, described as a "simple outpatient operation" whereby a surgeon "snips off the excess labia tissue with a small pair of surgical scissors," despite the out-of-pocket costs of between $1,500 and $3,000. Meyer also interviewed Antell, a New York cosmetic surgeon, who said "many women with oversize labia, like Dawn," complain their labia can be seen through pants or chafe when they walk. These complaints, however, were not the reason Dawn was considering the surgery, nor were they apparently the only reasons for which Antell performed the surgery: as Antell said, by "having her labia trimmed" it gave "a woman greater freedom and helps her feel better about her body and about herself in general" [38].

Meyer's article provided no evaluation of the procedure; indeed, in her critique of the article that appeared in *Ms.*, Rogan called Meyer's article a "free ad" for Antell, albeit one Rogan said misinformed its readers regarding typical labia and uncritically portrayed labiaplasty as a solution [39]. Some of the articles in the popular media were little short of announcements for the procedure and the clinicians – but they also indicate an uptake of labiaplasty by clinicians as an elective offering. The *Toronto Sun* in February 1999 told readers they no longer had to "fly to L.A. or New York to get the hottest trend in the world of cosmetic surgery – labiaplasty" as it was being offered "right here in T.O." The article provided information about the cost and length of labiaplasty [40]. Similarly, a 2011 article in *Jet* described the spa of a physician in Beverly Hills that included labiaplasty, described as a procedure that "trims the labia." And though noting cost could be high and recovery took six weeks, "for the many women who have issues with the appearance of their vagina," labiaplasty was "worth it to be comfortable in their skin" [41].

Popular print media covering labiaplasty were not always as glowing. A 1998 *Cosmopolitan* article, for example, discussed a woman who decided to "hop-on the latest, most controversial Hollywood plastic-surgery bandwagon" and have her labia surgically reduced. Though *Cosmopolitan* said labiaplasty "could actually work wonders," under a "Reality Check" subheading, it cautioned labiaplasty could remove skin, resulting in a "lessening of sensation." *Cosmopolitan* also noted because labiaplasty "is considered purely cosmetic" insurance would not cover the upwards of $3,000 cost, and the long recovery from swollen labia [42]. Indeed, *Cosmopolitan* – despite being focused on (hetero)sexual performance – in 2010 published an even more critical account of labiaplasty under the definitely not glowing title: "Vaginas Under Attack: Don't Let Greedy Gyno Talk You Into This Horrible Mistake" [43].

Though some labiaplasty practitioners complained that the media "in their quest for sensationalism frequently portrays labiaplasty as unnecessary and potentially dangerous" – as Hamori wrote regarding the 2010 *Cosmopolitan* article – these stories were sometimes driven by public relations agents for labiaplasty practitioners [31, 44]. But just because the story originated from a press release did not mean the resulting article was favorable. As an illustration, in 1998, reporter Kamps described her decision to follow up on what she described as a "curious press release" from Alter that encouraged women to "get out their hand mirrors" and examine their labia. Kamps considered this a joke – were "women really worrying about the size and shape of their labia" she wondered – so she interviewed Alter. Alter showed her before-and-after labiaplasty photographs. Kamps noted that though Alter "seems convinced there's something freakish about the [pre-surgery] women," she thought they looked normal. Indeed, she found the postoperative photographs to be "eerie" and "carbon copies of each other." After interviewing another surgeon who said the consequences of labiaplasty could be severe, Kamps

concluded by noting Alter failed to see how he was one of the people throwing out the so-called problem of what he deemed "labia envy" and that women "shouldn't catch the pitch" [45].

Regardless of the perspective on labiaplasty in the popular media, the articles educated readers about "labia envy" and provided the names of practitioners who offered labiaplasty. In that way, even the articles critical of labiaplasty were essentially free advertising for the surgery and its practitioners. As one industry newsletter noted: "the press has jumped on the bandwagon for labiaplasty, creating curiosity among women" [46]. This curiosity could arise even from articles not on the bandwagon.

But in addition to print media as effectively (if perhaps unintentionally) marketing labiaplasty, practitioners also said reality television shows focusing on cosmetic surgery increased awareness. These shows included the 2002 *Extreme Makeover*, and in 2004 *The Swan* and *Dr. 90201* [47]. In particular, practitioners pointed to Matlock's appearance on *Dr. 90210* and subsequent shows featuring labiaplasties [48]. Alter, who also appeared on *Dr. 90210*, said in 2007 that "[d]oing these procedures on a television show … makes people aware that they are available to them" and made labiaplasty "more acceptable" [49].

These shows could endlessly repeat and be shared on the internet, access to which began, by the late 1980s, to increase [50]. The advent and growth of the internet paralleled – and enabled – the growth of labiaplasty by allowing women, as a cosmetic surgery magazine noted in 2006, "to learn more in the privacy of their homes" [46]. Though in 2006 practitioners reported it was still more likely for patients to find them through word of mouth, it had become "more popular" for women to find out about them from the internet [46]. Women interviewed in 2006 indicated they initially found out about labiaplasty by doing searches for information on the internet, where they often found practitioners' websites [51, 52]. This trend of using the internet as a first means of gathering medical information only increased [53]. Searches were also done for cosmetic surgery: in one study, 95% of those surveyed said they used the internet to collect information about cosmetic surgery before seeing a clinician. This same study, however, found a "high percentage of poor quality internet sites," resulting in people coming away with "unrealistic expectations" created by the information they found on the internet [54].

Doing internet searches regarding labiaplasty easily led those seeking information to practitioner websites. A 2009 survey of ASPS members found that of the 750 (19.7% of members) who participated, a little more than half indicated they performed labiaplasty, and 18.9% advertised this surgery, with the internet being the most common method [55]. A 2012 study, however, found labiaplasty practitioners' websites provided no information about the diversity of female genitalia or regarding risks of labiaplasty [52].

Changes in Medical Practice

But it was not just the rise of lay access to information about female genitals and labiaplasty that enabled the surgery's growth: as others have noted, it was also changes in medical practice, in particular practitioners' capacity to market labiaplasty to women, that enabled the increase [56]. This ability to market themselves and procedures such as labiaplasty directly to patients was the result of a shift toward the commercialization of medicine. This shift began in 1982, when the Supreme Court ruled in favor of the Federal Trade Commission (FTC) against the American Medical Association (AMA), agreeing with the FTC that the AMA was in violation of antitrust laws by not allowing physicians to advertise beyond their type of practice and clinical hours [57]. Once considered part of the professional code of conduct to not directly solicit patients, in 1982 the AMA rewrote its ethical guidelines to remove restrictions "on advertising except those that can be specifically justified to protect the public from deceptive practices" [23, 57].

The removal of restrictions on advertising quickly led some physicians to begin promoting themselves in the local and national press as well as on billboards and through direct mail [57]. Though some older practitioners refrained from advertising, specialties that needed higher volumes of procedures like cosmetic surgery took it up [23]. Indeed, several cosmetic surgeons in California – despite the initial concerns of professional organizations against "hucksterism" – began advertising in the late 1970s [57].

This capacity to advertise cosmetic surgery paralleled an increased acceptance of it. While in the previous decades there had been stigma associated with cosmetic surgery, this perspective began to erode considerably in the 1970s, and cosmetic surgery moved from the margins of medicine to mainstream practice. This growing acceptance of cosmetic surgery as normative is illustrated by its appearance in women's popular magazines. In her examination, sociologist Sullivan found that cosmetic surgery was rarely covered before the 1980s: in the 1960s, only 15 articles about cosmetic surgery appeared and only 55 in the 1970s. By the 1980s, however, 107 articles appeared – though she thought this an underestimation, as it did not include the sex-and-body-focused *Cosmopolitan* [57]. Existing parallel, the number of cosmetic surgeries performed similarly grew, here in particular during the time labiaplasty started being electively offered: between 2000 and 2015, the ASPS reported a 115% increase in the number of cosmetic surgeries performed [58].

This dramatic increase in cosmetic surgeries was driven by physicians, Sullivan argued, who came to regard "appearance as a potential medical problem, conceptualize it in medical terms, and offer medical solutions." The physicians who performed cosmetic surgery often historically did so by justifying the surgery as a means of helping the mental health of their patients. But such a justification, Sullivan asserted, overlooks "the influence of the changing structural dimensions of the political economy of medicine, dimensions that also encourage[d] physicians to take up cosmetic surgery." Structural dimensions, according to Sullivan, included an increase in the number of physicians, especially ones in a surgical specialty, beginning in the 1980s. This growth encouraged physicians to specialize, including in cosmetic surgery, a specialty that saw an increase in practitioners by 269% – from 1,600 to 5,896 – between 1970 and 1996. The large growth in the number of cosmetic surgeons, combined with the fact that cosmetic surgery is a specialty defined by skill and not by anatomical location or disease state, meant surgeons began to worry about not only the increasing numbers in their own specialty but also competition for patients from other specialties offering cosmetic surgeries. This problem of a plethora of practitioners was furthered because of a reduction in the number of reconstructive, noncosmetic surgeries, meaning fewer cosmetic surgeons were needed to repair victims of, for example, car accident trauma, which had declined because of seat belts [57].

This decline in needed skills, but an increase of those with the skills, was compounded by, as Tomes outlined, a focus starting in the 1970s on cutting costs in medicine. By the 1980s, both public and private health care insurers in the United States began to set limits on what doctors and hospitals charged [23]. This led some physicians to offer services patients paid for directly, a point made by physician Norton when she said doctors were drawn to labiaplasty because they "just want something to supplement their income" [59]. In her article for *The Atlantic*, Myung-Ok Lee reported on the fifth annual Congress for Aesthetic Vaginal Surgery held in late 2010 and found more than one of the 60 attendees "groused" about poor insurance payments for things such as prenatal care and delivery compared to labiaplasty, which was a quick, in-office procedure with a cost of around $5,000 paid directly to them [48]. Or, as Matlock stated bluntly: "medicine is a business and sex is what sells" [46].

Running parallel to the increase in physician marketing following the FTC ruling and an uptake in the number of cosmetic surgeries was a move to regard the patient as a consumer of medicine. Medicine in the 1980s became increasingly corporate in ownership – of hospitals, of physician practices – and as part of this corporatization what historian Tomes described as a "recasting of the doctor–patient relationship" occurred, moving toward considering the parties involved as "providers and consumers." This drive to change the relationship was not solely the result of the corporate impetus in medicine; its origins can also be found in the rise of the patients' rights movements of the 1970s and of the move toward patient autonomy – and with it the capacity for patients to make informed choices about their health care – that also began in the 1970s and increased by the end of the century [23].

These structural changes led to, starting in the 1990s, a heightened competition among physicians to obtain paying patients for elective procedures. To attract such patients, cosmetic surgeons began to increase the number of procedures they offered beginning in the 1990s [57]. This increase included seeing an uncommon condition that rarely indicated surgery as being expandable to an offered one for patient consumption.

From an Emerging Trend to Mainstream Practice

FGCS practitioners suggest women "desire the youthful appearance of concealed labia minora and full smooth labia majora," [31] and that most "consider an aesthetic ideal a labia minora and clitoral hood that do not protrude past the labia majora" [29]. This, they assert, has resulted in "[i]ncreasing numbers of girls and young women" to seek "medical attention" [19]. Labiaplasty, as various practitioners have asserted, "has become a more commonly requested procedure by female patients" [60].

Clinicians once considered differently sized labia to be part of genital diversity, and labiaplasty only occasionally indicated. Clinical indications did not change between 1971 and 2017 – they have always involved comfort and appearance – yet the prevalence of labiaplasty increased. Practitioners commonly claim patients are driving this increase, this mainstreaming of the surgery. Such a claim, however, fails to acknowledge the parallel changes in medical practice that enabled FGCS practitioners to capitalize on the commercial potential of labiaplasty. The clinical indications did not change; but the economic ones did.

References

1. Oakes K. Is female genital cosmetic surgery going mainstream? *Ob Gyn News*. 2017. Available from: www .mdedge.com/obgynnews/article/141600/gynecology/female-genital-cosmetic-surgery-going-mainstream

2. American Society of Plastic Surgeons. Plastic Surgery Statistics Report 2016. Available from: www .plasticsurgery.org/documents/News/Statistics/2016/plastic-surgery-statistics-full-report-2016.pdf

3. Clerico C, Lari A, Mojallal A, Boucher F. Anatomy and aesthetics of the labia minora: The ideal vulva? *Aesth Plast Surg*. 2017;41:714–19.

4. ACOG 2017 Annual Clinical and Scientific Meeting. Expanding Cosmetic Gynecology Field Draws Concern. 2017. Available from: http://annualmeeting.acog.org /expanding-cosmetic-gynecology-field-draws-concern/ #.WaCAO5OGPq0

5. Runacres SA, Wood PL. Cosmetic labiaplasty in an adolescent population. *J Pediatr Adolesc Gynecol*. 2016;29:218–22.

6. Essen B, Johnsdotter S. Female genital mutilation in the West: Traditional circumcision versus genital cosmetic surgery. *Acta Obstet Gynecol Scand*. 2004;83:611–13.

7. Hodgkinson DJ, Hait G. Aesthetic vaginal labioplasty. *Plast Reconstr Surg*. 1984;74:414–16.

8. Oranges CM, Sisti A, Sisti G. Labia minora reduction techniques: A comprehensive literature review. *Aesthet Surg J*. 2015;35:419–31.

9. Bates B. Controversy rages over female genital cosmetic surgery. *Ob Gyn News*. March 2010:1.

10. Capraro VJ. Congenital anomalies. *Clin Obstet Gynecol.* 1971;14:988–1012.

11. Rouzier R, Louis-Sylvestre C, Paniel BJ, et al. Hypertrophy of labia minora: Experience with 163 reductions. *Am J Obstet Gynecol.* 2000;182:35–40.

12. Gowen RM, Martin VL. Labia minora reduction in an iron-lung disabled woman. *Obstet Gynecol.* 1988;71:488–9.

13. Chavis, WM, LaFerla JJ, Niccolini R. Plastic repair of elongated, hypertrophic labia minora. *J Reprod Med.* 1989;34:373–5.

14. Fliegner JRH. Vulval varicosities and labial reduction. *Aust N Z J Obstet Gynecol.* 1997;37:129–30.

15. Maas SM, Hage JJ. Functional and aesthetic labia minora reduction. *Plast Reconstr Surg.* 2000;105:1453–6.

16. Sakamoto H, Ichikawa G, Shimizu Y, et al. Extreme hypertrophy of the labia minora. *Acta Obstet Gynecol Scand.* 2004;83:1225–6.

17. Lynch A, Marulaiah M, Samarakkody U. Reduction labioplasty in adolescents. *J Pediatr Adolesc Gynecol.* 2008;21:147–9.

18. Triana L, Robledo AM. Refreshing labioplasty techniques for plastic surgeons. *Aesth Plast Surg.* 2012;26:1078–86.

19. Reddy J, Laufer MR. Hypertrophic labia minora. *J Pediatr Adolesc Gynecol.* 2010; 23:3–6.

20. Cao YJ, Li FY, Li SK, et al. A modified method of labia minora reduction: The de-epithelialised reduction of the central and posterior labia minora. *J Plast Reconstr Aesthet Surg.* 2012;65:1096–102.

21. Lista F, Bhavik D, Mistry BD, et al. The safety of aesthetic labiaplasty: A plastic surgery experience. *Aesthet Surg J.* 2015;35:689–95.

22. Solanki NS, Tejero-Trujeque R, Stevens-King A, et al. Aesthetic and functional reduction of the labia minora using the Maas and Hage technique. *J Plast Reconstr Aesthet Surg.* 2010;63:1181–5.

23. Tomes N. *Remaking the American patient: How Madison Avenue and modern medicine turned patients into consumers.* Chapel Hill: University of North Carolina Press; 2016.

24. Radman HM. Hypertrophy of the labia minora. *Obstet Gynecol.* 1976;48:78s–80s.

25. Honoré LH, O'Hara KE. Benign enlargement of the labia minora: Report of two cases. *Eur J Obstet Gynecol Reprod Biol.* 1978;8:61–4.

26. Laufer MR, Galvin WJ. Labial hypertrophy: A new surgical approach. *Adolesc Pediatr Gynecol.* 1995;8:39–41.

27. Munhoz AM, Filassi JR, Ricci MD, et al. Aesthetic labia minora reduction with inferior wedge resection and superior pedicle flap reconstruction. *Plast Reconstr Surg.* 2006;118:1237–47.

28. Alter GJ. A new technique for aesthetic labia minora reduction. *Ann Plast Surg.* 1998;40:287–90.

29. Alter GJ. Aesthetic labia minora and clitoral hood reduction using extended central wedge resection. *Plast Reconstr Surg.* 2008;122:1780–9.

30. Lewis W. The shape of things to come: The risks and rewards of vaginal aesthetic surgery. *Plast Surg Pract.* 2008;January:30–3.

31. Hamori CA. Aesthetic surgery of the female genitalia: Labiaplasty and beyond. *Plast Reconstr Surg.* 2014;134:661–73.

32. Bramwell R. Invisible labia: The representation of female external genitals in women's magazines. *Sex Relat Ther.* 2002;17:187–90.

33. Kobrin S. More women seek vaginal plastic surgery. Womens eNews. November 14, 2004.

34. Doup L. Women choosing genital plastic surgery. *South Bend Tribune.* June 8, 2005.

35. Placik OJ, Arkins JP. Plastic surgery trends parallel *Playboy* magazine: The pudenda preoccupation. *Aesthet Surg J.* 2014;34:1083–90.

36. Schick VR, Rima BN, Calabrese SK. Evulvalution: The portrayal of women's external genitalia and physique across time and current Barbie doll ideals. *J Sex Res.* 2011;48:74–81.

37. Kelishadi SS, Elston JB, Rao AJ, et al. Posterior wedge resection: A more aesthetic labiaplasty. *Aesthet Surg J.* 2013;33:847–53.

38. Meyer C. The big report: Intimate surgery. *For Women First.* August 1, 1994.

39. Rogan H. A women's mag masks sleaze as service. *Ms.* September/October 1994.

40. Stapells C. 'Designer vaginas' available in Toronto. *Toronto Sun*, February 5, 1999.

41. Turner M. 'V' is for vanity. *Jet.* September 12, 2011.

42. Havranek C. The new sex surgeries. *Cosmopolitan.* November 1998.

43. Triffin M. Vaginas under attack: Don't let greedy gyno talk you into this horrible mistake. *Cosmopolitan.* July 2010.

44. Braun V. Female genital cosmetic surgery: A critical review of current knowledge and contemporary debates. *J Womens Health.* 2010;19:1393–407.

45. Kamps L. Labia envy. Salon.Com, March 17, 1998.

46. Ranft L. Something to talk about. Plastic Surgery ProductsOnline.com, November 2006.

47. Tiefer L. Female genital cosmetic surgery: Freakish or inevitable? Analysis from medical marketing,

bioethics, and feminist theory. *Feminism Psychol.* 2008;18:466–79.

48. Lee MM-O. Perverse incentives: Gynecologists cash in on an intimate new market. *The Atlantic.* June 2011.

49. Perrine JW. Surgery where? *Self.* September 23, 2007.

50. Moschovitis CJP, Poole H, Schuyler T, et al. History of the Internet: A chronology, 1843 to the present. Santa Barbara: ABC-CLIO, 1999.

51. Spivak T. "In the pink." HoustonPress.Com, May 11, 2006. Available from: www.houstonpress.com/news/in-the-pink-6546280

52. Liao L-M, Taghinejadi N, Creighton SM. An analysis of the content and clinical implications of online advertisements for female genital cosmetic surgery. *BMJ Open.* 2012;2:e001908.

53. Fox S, Duggan M. Health Online 2013. Pew Research Center. 2013. Available from: www.pewinternet.org/2013/01/15/health-online-2013/

54. Montemurro P, Porcnik A, Heden P, et al. The influence of social media and easily accessible online information on the aesthetic plastic surgery practice: Literature review and our own experience. *Aesth Plast Surg.* 2015;39: 270–7.

55. Mirzabeii MN, Moore JH, Mericli AF, et al. Current trends in vaginal labioplasty. *Ann Plast Surg.* 2012;68: 125–34.

56. Braun V. In search of (better) sexual pleasure: Female genital 'cosmetic' surgery. *Sexualities* 2005;8:407–24.

57. Sullivan DA. *Cosmetic medicine: The cutting edge of commercial medicine in America.* New Brunswick, NJ: Rutgers University Press; 2001.

58. American Society of Plastic Surgeons. New statistics reflect the changing face of plastic surgery. 2016. Available from: www.plasticsurgery.org/news/press-releases/new-statistics-reflect-the-changing-face-of-plastic-surgery

59. Scheeres J. Vulva goldmine: How cosmetic surgeons snatch your money. Bitch. May 31, 2000.

60. Gonzalez F, Dass D, Almeida B. Custom flask labiaplasty. *Aesthet Surg J.* 2015;75:266–71.

Techniques of Female Genital Cosmetic Surgery

Angelica Kavouni Ion and Sarah M. Creighton

Introduction

Female cosmetic genital surgery (FGCS), sometimes referred to as vaginal rejuvenation, is an umbrella term encompassing multiple plastic surgery procedures that are quite distinct from one another but are often used in combination to achieve a certain vulval appearance. The procedures are performed across several surgical specialties, including urology, gynaecology and plastic surgery. Numerous FGCS techniques are on offer and surgeons may also adapt standard techniques to better suit differences in genital anatomy and satisfy patient requests. Most procedures are operations to alter the external genital appearance, although procedures to tighten the vagina may also be requested and can be performed at the same time. Labiaplasty is the most frequently performed operation on the external genitalia and has become synonymous with cosmetic surgery of the female genitalia. It would be impossible to describe all FGCS procedures in a single chapter. This chapter focuses on labiaplasty techniques.

Normal female genital anatomy is described in detail elsewhere (Chapter 2 by Crouch, this volume). Although there is a wide variation in the normal width of the labia minora and, to some extent, the labia majora, patients who express concerns to surgeons usually complain that the labia minora are too large. Surgeons often describe this as 'labial hypertrophy', although this has not been well defined and may well describe normally sized labia. There is no underlying medical cause for labial hypertrophy. Women requesting surgery usually desire a prepubescent aesthetic. The labia majora of young females tend to be fuller and smoother and nearly approximate in the midline just in front of the clitoris to form the intervulvar commissure on the standing position. To achieve this aesthetic, which is associated with younger age, the labia minora are reduced sufficiently to be hidden behind the symmetrical labia majora, giving the vulva a smoother, 'clamshell' appearance without unwanted tissue [1] (Figure 5.1a and b). Some patients will express concerns about their clitoral hood in addition to labial concerns. They may complain about unwanted skin

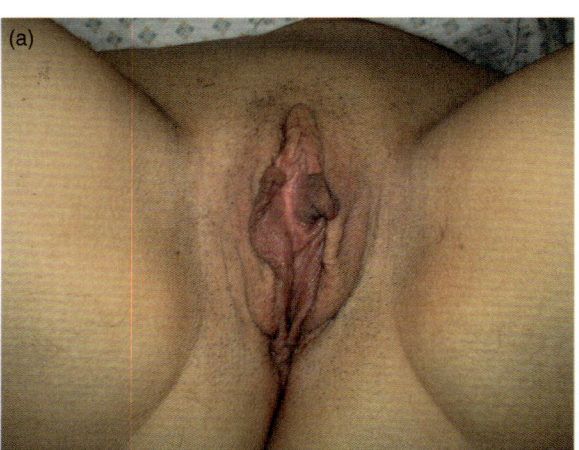
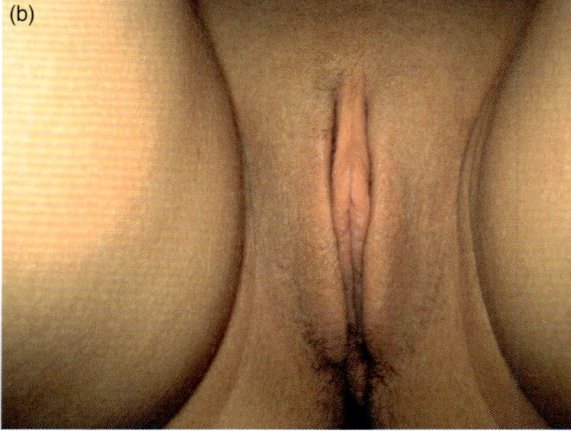

Figure 5.1 (a) Preoperative picture of patient requesting labial reduction for perceived excessive labia minora. (b) The same patient after labiaplasty perfomed with labial trimming technique.

folds of the clitoral hood as well as any perceived wrinkling and/or protrusion. There is a wide age range for patients requesting labiaplasty, with reports in the literature ranging from 16 to 68 years [2]. Only a few articles report preoperative width, but where it is recorded the average width measured from midline to the lateral edge of the labia minora ranges from 2.7 to 5 cm. Because of the wide variation in perineal anatomy and the high incidence of asymmetry, meeting the patient's cosmetic goals can be challenging. A thorough assessment is therefore crucial, even if it involves several consultations.

Before the Operation

Physical examination of the patient has two purposes:

- To exclude any underlying pathology which may be causing or exacerbating vulval symptoms
- To assess specific vulval concerns and plan appropriate cosmetic genital surgery

Physical Examination to Exclude Underlying Pathology

In a small proportion of cases there will be a medical cause for perceived labial enlargement, and a careful medical examination of the genitals is essential. It is important to exclude rare causes, such as androgenic hormones, either exogenous or as a result of a virilising medical condition, and sensitivity to topical oestrogen. Stretching or weight attachment of the labia for sexual enhancement or as female genital mutilation will lengthen the labia. Dermatitis (which can be secondary to urinary incontinence) and vulvar lymphedema (swelling either post cancer radiation or as a primary disease) must be excluded. It is important to evaluate genital skin health and note conditions such as lichen sclerosus (irregular silver plaques) and herpes simplex lesions (grouped vesicles/blisters). Symptoms such as urinary tract and vaginal infections, urinary incontinence and prolapse may exacerbate labial discomfort, and in some cases referral to a urogynaecologist may be indicated.

Fat loss associated with age, menopause and weight loss can result in flattening of the mons pubis and the labia majora. This can create a perception of excess labia majora skin. Palpation of the clitoris is important to rule out clitoral enlargement as the cause of the prominent appearance of the clitoral hood. Any current or previous medical or psychological problems must be documented and investigated appropriately. Smoking is thought to have a detrimental impact on labial healing after surgery and smoking cessation advice should be offered. It is useful to ask about other lifestyle factors that are potentially implicated in labial health such as hygiene.

Physical Examination to Plan Surgery

Once any underlying pathology is ruled out, the second part of the physical examination is to decide if surgery is indicated and, if so, which technique is most likely to meet expectations. The contour changes of the labia and any vaginal tears resulting from childbirth or injuries should be recorded. Physical examination of the vulva should assess the extent of both vertical and horizontal skin excess and the presence of asymmetry. The amount of subcutaneous fat is evaluated and the skin checked for elasticity and signs of atrophy. The overall pattern of skin and fat distribution in the labia should be noted as well as the presence and extent of any varicosities (prominent veins). The presence and shape of clitoral hood folds and the condition of the hymen or its remnants should be noted. The examination should be performed both in the supine and standing positions.

Preoperative photographs in both the standing and lithotomy positions are usually taken for all cosmetic perineal procedures. Patients frequently do not look at themselves carefully with a mirror in lithotomy position (lying down with legs apart) before the operation, as they are primarily concerned with the standing view. However, postoperatively, they may then notice pre-existing irregularities for the first time.

The decision to proceed with labia minor and /or labia majora surgery is primarily guided by the extent of the patient's desire to change. It is best that the patient demonstrates a clear understanding of the limitations of labia minora and majora contouring to avoid postoperative disappointment. The risks and benefits for each method should be discussed with patients and the technique used should be based on patient anatomy and patient preference weighted with the desired appearance outcome.

Agreeing on the Goals of Surgery

While the most frequently expressed goal for patients seeking labiaplasty is simply to make the labia minora smaller and/or eliminate significant asymmetry, surgery is often more complex than simple excision.

Surgeons see the goal of labiaplasty as aligning as far as possible the patient's existing external genital to the most desirable appearance in our contemporary world. This aesthetic is based on a differently balanced relationship between the labia minora, clitoral hood and the labia majora. To achieve this balance, the surgeon must address this three-dimensional problem with a series of steps that involve reducing the excess skin and redistributing the fat tissue in a three-dimensional fashion. Clitoral hood contour and clitoral hood ptosis (drooping) may pose a significant challenge and contribute to a 'top heavy' appearance. Reducing clitoral hood folds and skin advancement flaps (moving small sections of skin to a different position in the vulva) may be employed to avoid this outcome. It is essential to maintain the neurovascular (blood and nerve) supply to the skin and to preserve the vaginal introitus (entrance) as well as achieving an optimal color/texture match.

For patients who have experienced deflation of the volume of the labia majora due to either weight loss or natural ageing, revolumising of the area using fat transfer techniques can create fuller shaped outer labia. It may be combined with minor skin reduction of the labia major and radio frequency skin tightening. Pubic mound contour should be kept in mind when planning labia majora augmentation to avoid a mismatch. It is often useful to combine lipocontouring (using ultrasound to reduce localized fat) of the pubic mound to achieve the desired vulva aesthetic.

Finally, it is important to clarify whether the patient is seeking surgery for purely aesthetic or functional reasons or with the hope of enhancing sexual satisfaction. An inquiry as to the status of sexual function among women seeking surgery is therefore necessary. It is important to ensure that the patients understand that surgery of the vulval area is not meant to improve a person's sex life. Informed consent for elective procedures such as labiaplasty and other FGCS procedures should always include a detailed exploration with the patient of the option of no intervention; a 'cool-off' period is crucial [3].

Current Surgical Techniques

The history and clinical outcomes of labiaplasty are described in Chapter 6 by Michala and Chapter 4 by Rodriguez (this volume). Since the inception of labiaplasty into the plastic surgery literature by Hodgkinson and Hait in 1984 [4], there have been multiple new technique introductions and modifications. Surgical techniques that have been reported in the literature since that article was published include de-epithelialisation, direct excision, W-shaped resection, wedge resection, composite reduction, Z-plasty and laser labiaplasty [5]. Each labiaplasty technique offers its own advantages and disadvantages. Unfortunately, in the literature to date there is an absence of comparative analysis of the reported labiaplasty techniques to establish criteria for operative planning.

In general the term labiaplasty refers to reduction of the size of the labia minora. Less commonly, however, labia majora reduction is sometimes performed. Conversely, on occasion reduction of the labia minor may be combined with techniques such as fat injection to plump up the labia majora to achieve a more youthful genital contour. There are several main surgical approaches to labiaplasty. Each approach has its own advantages and disadvantages. Surgeons may use a combination of techniques or modify a technique depending on the final outcome which they and the patient hope to achieve.

Labiaplasty of the Labia Minora

The following are broad descriptions of the types of surgical techniques which may be used in labiaplasty of the labia minora.

Labia Minora Excision (Resection, Trim)

The labia minora can be directly excised by trimming a strip of skin from the lateral aspect (outside edge) of each labia [6] (Figure 5.2a). This procedure is the most straightforward technique and is probably more commonly performed by gynaecologists than cosmetic plastic surgeons. Direct labial excision provides a simple way for the excision of excess tissue, as requested by many patients. This technique, however, removes the natural contour, colour and texture of the free edge of the labia minora. It places a suture line at the free edge of the labia minora, which may lead to visible scar formation (Figure 5.2b). A 'dog-ear' (a corner of skin which is more prominent) can be formed at the edge of the incision nearest to the clitoris and can look unsightly. Sensation may, in theory, be affected by scar formation along the border of the labia minora, although neither of these statements regarding scar formation has been validated in any study thus far.

Labial trimming

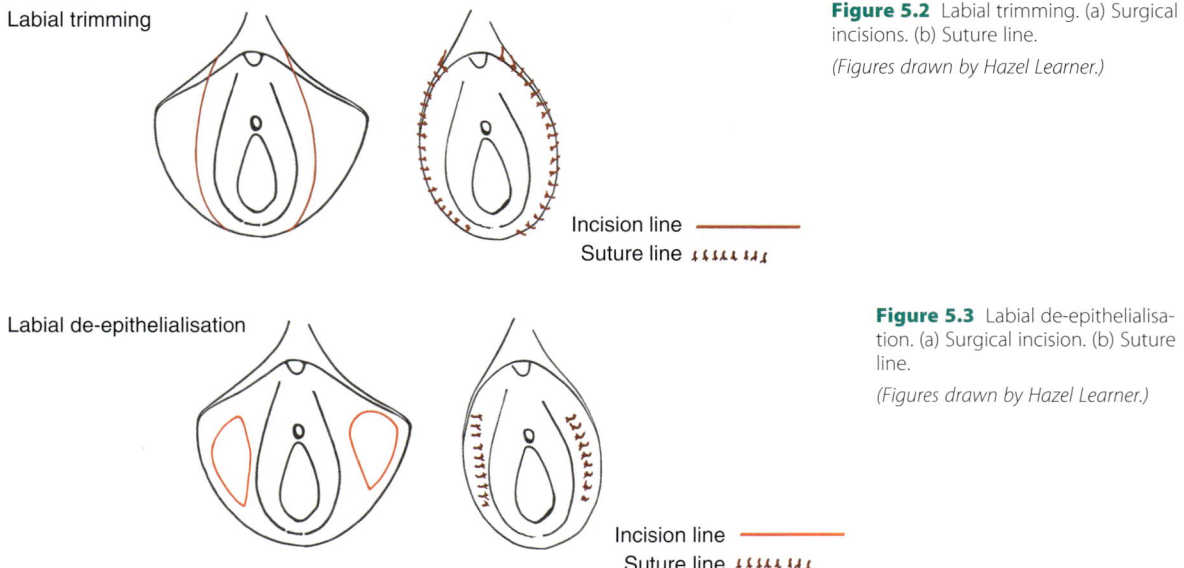

Figure 5.2 Labial trimming. (a) Surgical incisions. (b) Suture line.

(Figures drawn by Hazel Learner.)

Incision line ———
Suture line ⨪⨪⨪⨪

Labial de-epithelialisation

Figure 5.3 Labial de-epithelialisation. (a) Surgical incision. (b) Suture line.

(Figures drawn by Hazel Learner.)

Incision line ———
Suture line ⨪⨪⨪⨪

De-epitheliasation

In de-epithelialisation techniques, an oval area of skin on the central and lateral (outside) edges of the labial minora is identified and marked. The overlying skin (epithelium) is removed while preserving the underlying tissues. The skin edges of this area are then stitched together (Figure 5.3a). The advantages of this type of surgery are that it preserves the natural outside border of the labia minora and the neurovascular (blood and nerve) supply [7]. In all studies of the de-epithelialisation technique, complications are few. However, this technique may not work as well in patients with wider labia, as it may not reduce enough tissue bulk. The scar is in the middle of the labia (Figure 5.3b) and may leave the centre of each labia with an uneven appearance.

Wedge Resection

A V-shaped wedge of skin is excised from the most protuberant part of the labia minora (Figure 5.4a). The cut edges are then stitched together, leaving the free border of the reduced labia without an exposed scar. The scar runs at right angles to the free edge of the labia (Figure 5.4b). The angle, exact placement and extent of the wedge resection will vary depending on the quantity of tissue excess and the degree of skin laxity. Wedge resection also retains the natural contour and colour of the free edge of the labia minora. However, this technique may create an abrupt contrast in the colour of the labia minora where tissues are stitched together [8].

Some surgeons have argued that the longitudinal scar created by this technique may distort the labia, creating a depression at the point of the scar, but this concern has not been validated.

Composite Reduction

Composite reduction is a technique that addresses both labial protrusion and clitoral hooding, and excellent aesthetic outcomes have been reported [9]. As opposed to other procedures that are based on reducing just the part of the labia minora below the clitoris, the composite procedure also entails removal of tissue located to the side of and above the clitoris. This creates separate segments positioned in a way that enables uniform reduction of the labia across their entire length, especially in the clitoral hood area. Reports of overall patient satisfaction is high and an improvement of sexual excitability has been observed in approximately 35% of the cases [9]. This may possibly be due to the clitoris being positioned closer to the vaginal introitus resulting in more direct clitoral stimulation during intercourse.

W-Shaped Resection and Z-Plasty

W-shaped resection and Z-plasty have been described in only a handful of patients. These techniques use different incisions on the labia – the cuts are made in the shape of the letter W or Z. Closure of the opposing W-shaped incisions results in a zigzag suture line

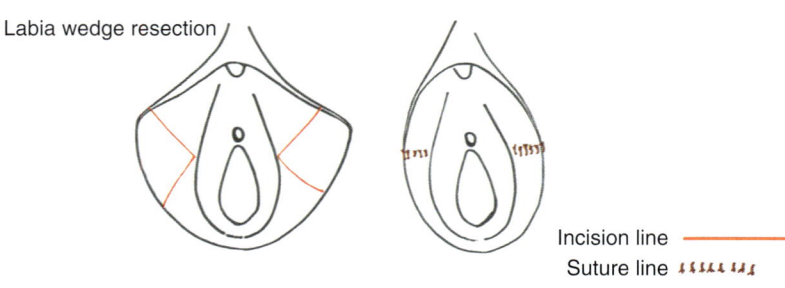

Labia wedge resection

Figure 5.4 Wedge resection. (a) Surgical incision. (b) Suture line.
(Figures drawn by Hazel Learner.)

Incision line ———
Suture line ⟋⟋⟋⟋⟋ ⟋⟋⟋

running obliquely across the edge of the labium with minimal tension. Advantages of this technique are thought to be less wound dehiscence (wound separation) and advancement (bringing forward) of the posterior fourchette (back edge of the vaginal entrance).

Laser Labiaplasty

Laser labiaplasty is a surgical procedure in which an ablative laser is used to perform either direct excision or wedge resection, effectively replacing the use of scalpel or scissors.

Selecting the Surgical Techniques

A wide variation in genital anatomy exists, as described in detail in Chapter 2 by Crouch (this volume). Surgeons have proposed several systems in order to stage the degree of labial hypertrophy in an attempt to standardise the choice of operation. Currently, however, there is no consensus on how best to define and classify labial hypertrophy. The most widely used classification system was first described by Franco in 1993 [10] and divides labial hypertrophy into four stages using the width of the labia minora: stage I – less than 2 cm; stage II – 2 to 4 cm; stage III – 4 to 6 cm; and stage IV – greater than 6 cm. The distance is measured in centimetres from the base of the labia minora (at the vaginal introitus) to the distal most point of the labia minora tip. Some surgical studies suggested an algorithm pairing the degree or shape of hypertrophy with the optimal surgical procedure. For example, Ellsworth et al. [11] suggested that patients with Franco type I and type II labia minora hypertrophy may be treated most effectively with the de-epithelialisation technique. Patients with Franco type III or type IV labia minora hypertrophy may be less appropriate candidates for the de-epithelialisation technique because of inability to reduce labial volume completely and poor aesthetic outcomes. Instead, these patients may be more suitable candidates for either the direct excision or the

wedge resection technique. Needless to say, there is no evidence base to support these recommendations. Surgeons will in general choose the techniques with which they are the most familiar and that reliably produce outcomes that they and their patients are happy with.

Operative Approaches

The following section describes some general surgical principles and includes some examples of the more commonly used techniques in FGCS. The scope of this chapter does not give space for an extensive description. Interested readers will find more detailed surgical description in a surgical atlas.

The following procedures are described:

1. Wedge resection of labia minora
2. Reduction of the labia majora
3. Revolumising of labia majora
4. Clitoral hood reduction

General Principles

Anaesthesia and Antibiotics

If the patient is undergoing labiaplasty only, then this is commonly performed with local anaesthesia administered with anxiolytic medicines and monitored anaesthesia care. General (full) anaesthesia is used for patients undergoing more than one concurrent procedure. Intraoperative antibiotics are often recommended and these would usually be broad-spectrum antibiotics such as cefazolin or cefotaxime and metronidazole.

Positioning and Skin Marking

The patient is placed in the lithotomy (legs up) position in stirrups to support the calf and foot. If the procedure is performed with local anaesthetic, the patient can choose to hold a hand mirror to review her genitalia while she is positioned in stirrups as the surgeon discusses both her anatomy and the procedure. The surgeon will mark the proposed skin incisions with a non-indelible pen to plan the wedge of labial tissue to be removed (Figure 5.5). When planning the wedge, it is important that the tissue is removed from the most protuberant portion of the labia minora. It is also important to avoid removing too large a wedge, as the edges of the labial defect should close with minimal tension.

Closing the Wounds

The type of suture (stitch) used to close the wounds varies greatly. The most commonly used sutures are soluble (dissolving) sutures. The technique of the closure may vary according to the surgeon's preference; either continuous (one long stitch under the skin edge) or interrupted (separate) sutures may be used.

Wedge Resection of Labia Minora

The wedge resection may be performed either with the scalpel (knife), scissors, radio frequency (high-frequency current) or laser. The frenulum is a small fold of skin at the base of the clitoris where the two labia minora meet and is a good landmark to start marking the incision. Surgeons will avoid cutting the frenulum itself, as it can heal with some thickening and a bulbous (lumpy) appearance. Using a sterile marker pen, the surgeon marks a gentle arc from the

frenulum to the posterior (back) end of the labia minora. A scalpel is most commonly used to make the incisions and needlepoint electrocautery (electrical current) is used to remove the wedge. It is recommended to maintain some submucosa (tissue underlying the outer layer of skin) along each edge. In particular, in patients with atrophic and thin labia minora, it is best to de-mucosalise (remove just the outer layer of skin of) the wedge rather than perform a full-thickness resection. It is important to make sure all bleeding is controlled to reduce the risk of bleeding and haematoma (bruising). If a 'dog-ear' (a corner of skin which is more prominent) is formed laterally, a narrow triangle of labia minora skin above the 'dog-ear' can be removed which will leave the scar along the interlabial groove (skin crease) which is less noticeable. A modification of the wedge technique with a lateral 'hockey-stick' incision to address minor clitoral hood redundancy has been described [12]. Attention is paid in order to preserve sufficient labia length while also incorporating suture techniques that promote smooth, flat scars and avoid wavy edges.

Reduction of the Labia Majora

Preparation, anaesthesia and skin marking are performed as described earlier.

Labia majora reduction is usually performed through an incision (cut) running front to back on the inside of the redundant labia majora. The incision should be placed just lateral (outside) to the junction of the hair-bearing labia majora skin and the smooth skin of the intervulvar cleft. This placement prevents the transfer of the hair-bearing skin to the edge of the vagina, which may be a source of irritation. It is important not to remove too much tissue to prevent pulling and resultant splaying open of the labia minora because of lateral tension.

The skin markings are performed based on the amount of tissue excess. If there is only moderate tissue excess, an ellipse of skin may be removed as one continuous segment on either side of the labia majora. If there is significant laxity and multiple folds of the majora are present as, for example, in patients after massive weight loss, then the medial (inner) incision should be made first. The labia majora skin flap are lifted up medially to laterally (centre to edge) with the help of wide double skin hooks and using point tip cautery. The underlying fatty tissue may be removed if necessary to reduce the bulk of the refashioned labia majora.

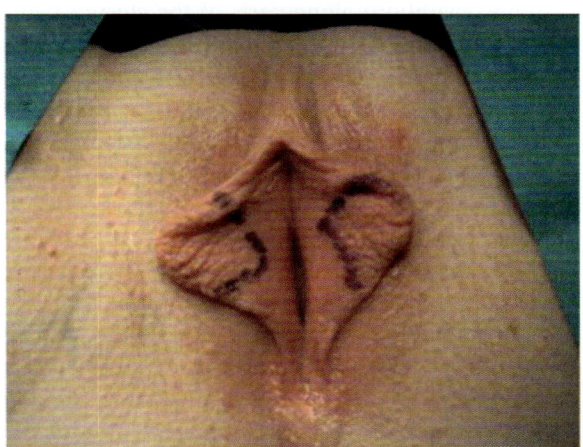

Figure 5.5 Photograph of skin markings prior to excision of wedge of labial tissue.

Revolumising of Labia Majora

Revolumising of labia majora can be done at the same time as labia minora reduction and involves fat injection into the mons pubis and/or the labia majora. If the patient requires fat transfer to the labia majora, this may be performed in the lithotomy (legs up) position to facilitate access to various fat donor sites such as the abdomen, flanks and outer thighs. The average fat harvest for fat grafting of these areas is approximately 100 cc. Depending on the amount of deflation that is present and the patient preference, the mons pubis may be injected with 20 cc of fat and each labia majora may be injected with 10 cc. Overfilling of the areas may be necessary by 20% to 30% to account for fat loss in the following 6 to 9 months. It is recommended to inject the mons pubis first to allow for elongation and elevation of the labia majora anteriorly. Then the labia majora themselves are injected. Conservative filling of the labia majora is important to avoid creating bulk. If there is widening of the intervulvar commissure or cleft, one may consider grafting the superomedial portion of the labia majora in order to approximate the cleft and attempt to conceal somewhat the prominent clitoral hood.

Clitoral Hood Reduction

Excess skin folds of the clitoral hood can be addressed by removing an ellipse of skin. Markings are performed before making an inverted V-type incision and removing excess skin while preventing exposure of the glans clitoris. Reduction of skin on either side of the clitoris may be performed by removing two triangles of skin along each side of the clitoral hood. The excision is performed preferably with a scalpel, and following excision meticulous care must be taken to stop all bleeding. The depth of the excision should be kept very superficial to avoid injury of the dorsal clitoral nerve which lies under the investing fascia (a sheet of stronger skin) around the clitoris.

Postoperative Care

Topical or oral antibiotics are recommended for 3 to 5 days after the procedure. Patients are instructed to reduce activity to a minimum for a week, during which they may put ice packs on the vulva and elevate their pelvis on pillows while they lie down. They can urinate in the shower or while pouring water from a jug when on the toilet. In general, avoidance of bathtubs, tampons and sexual activity is recommended for 3 to 4 weeks. Meticulous perineal hygiene and dressing with a sterile pad and use of anti-inflammatory drugs and other analgesics for postoperative pain and inflammation are also recommended. Activities such as cycling may be resumed after 6 weeks and horseback riding after 12 weeks. Post-operative swelling, especially of the labia minora edge, can last 3 to 6 months.

Complications

Postoperative complications include wound dehiscence (wound separation), haematoma formation (bruising), recurrent bleeding from the wound edges, flap necrosis (death of labial skin after wedge resection), discomfort, visible scarring, superficial infections, under-resection (not enough skin removed) and over-resection (too much skin removed) [13]. Suture granulomas (inflammation around a stitch), fistula formation (button holes in the labia) and a clitoral hood 'dog-ear' are rarer complications.

The most common complications are edge separations or stretching of the labium. Another complication seen with wedge labiaplasty is a mismatch of the pigmentation along the arch of the labia minora causing a prominent stripe between dark and lighter parts of the labia minora. This may be prevented by positioning the wedge within the pigmented portion of the labia minora. Notching (pulling in) of the labia minor edge can occur if the wound edges are not properly everted (positioned during suturing) [14]. Dehiscence (wound separation) along parts of the closure (windows or partial gaps) seems to be more common in smokers undergoing wedge labiaplasty or if excess submucosa is removed in the wedge. In general, as much submucosa should be left behind as possible. The only exception to this would be in very thick labia minora, where reduction of the bulk helps the overall aesthetic result [15, 16].

Labia majora labiaplasty scars are located in the interlabial groove (skin crease) but are more visible than labia minora labiaplasty scars on lithotomy view (legs apart). Over-resection of the labia majora (removing too much skin) may cause scar thickening or scar overgrowth (hypertrophy), flattening of the appearance of the labia majora and further visibility of the scar. The scar is best placed along the medial (inside) border of the labia majora (sagittal hairline) to preserve the hairless skin separating the majora and the minora. This modification prevents the placing of hair-bearing skin adjacent to the vaginal opening which might be a potential source of painful sexual intercourse.

Scars from clitoral hood reduction may hypertrophy (overgrow) and contract (tighten), thus exposing the clitoris. This may prove a most challenging complication and may be addressed with revision surgery using labia minora transposition flaps.

The Role of Adjunctive Treatments

Non-surgical reduction of the labia majora may be performed with radio frequency devices. The thermal energy is used to denature the dermal collagen and induce remodeling and tissue tightening. Usually only mild skin redundancy may be improved with the use of radio frequency energy. The procedure is performed every 4 to 6 weeks for three or four sessions and the results are evident after 6 to 9 months.

Revision Labiaplasty

A proportion of women will be unhappy with the results of their labiaplasty and may seek further genital surgery. The actual numbers of women seeking revision surgery is unknown but increasing numbers of clinics now advertise revision procedures for what is often termed 'botched labiaplasty'. There is little information on the surgical approaches required to address women's concerns and more research is needed.

Conclusion

Labiaplasty of the labia minora is by far the most frequently performed cosmetic operation on the female genitalia. Despite its popularity, current practices remain poorly described, with a lack of standardisation and no uniformity in practice [17]. This makes it impossible to evaluate a particular technique on a large enough number of patients across treatment services and follow them up. There are therefore few prospective clinical studies on labiaplasty and no evidence-based guidance. It is all the more important that surgeons offering labiaplasty undertake a careful clinical assessment and ensure patients have taken on board the known benefits and risks of the intervention as well as what is not known. Informed consent for elective procedure should always include discussion with the patient of the option of no intervention. Clear communication over time is required to ascertain that the consenting patient has realistic expectations of what can be achieved to avoid postoperative disappointment and the possibility of further surgery. Until comparative studies become available, the best techniques will remain the ones the surgeon is most comfortable with and which achieve consistent results.

References

1. Clerico C, Lari T, Mojallal A, et al. Anatomy and aesthetics of the labia minora: The ideal vulva? *Aesth Plast Surg.* 2017;41:714–19.

2. Radman HM. Hypertrophy of the labia minora. *Obstet Gynecol.* 1976;48(Suppl):78S–79S.

3. Liao LM, Chadwick PM, Tamar-Mattis A. Informed consent in pediatric and adolescent gynecology: From ethical principles to ethical behavior. In Creighton SM, Balen A, Breech L, Liao LM (eds), *Pediatric and adolescent gynecology: A problem-based approach.* Cambridge: Cambridge University Press; 2018.

4. Hodgkinson DJ, Hait G. Aesthetic vaginal labioplasty. *Plast Reconstr Surg.* 1984;74:414–16.

5. Felicio Yde A. Labial surgery. *Aesthet Surg J.* 2007;27:322–8.

6. Furnas HJ. Trim labiaplasty. *Plast Reconstr Surg Glob Open.* 2017;5(5):e1349.

7. Choi HY, Kim KT. A new method for aesthetic reduction of labia minora (the deepithelialized reduction of labioplasty). *Plast Reconstr Surg.* 2000;105:419–22; discussion 423–4.

8. Alter GJ. A new technique for aesthetic labia minora reduction. *Ann Plast Surg.* 1998;40:287–90.

9. Gress S. Composite reduction labiaplasty. *Aesth Plast Surg.* 2013;37:674–83.

10. Franco T, Franco D, Hipertrofia de ninfas. *J Bras Ginecol.* 1993 103(5):163–5.

11. Ellsworth WA, Rizvi M, Lypka M, et al. Techniques for labia minora reduction: An algorithmic approach. *Aesth Plast Surg.* 2010;34:105–10.

12. Alter GJ. Aesthetic labia minora and clitoral hood reduction using extended central wedge resection. *Plast Reconstr Surg.* 2008;122:1780–9.

13. Alter GJ. Labia minora reconstruction using clitoral hood flaps, wedge excisions, and YV

advancement flaps. *Plast Reconstr Surg.* 2011;127:2356–63.

14. Hamori CA. Aesthetic surgery of the female genitalia: Labiaplasty and beyond. *Plast Reconstr Surg.* 2014;134:661–73.

15. Lista F, Mistry BD, Singh Y, et al. The safety of aesthetic labiaplasty: A plastic surgery experience. *Aesthet Surg J.* 2015;35:689–95.

16. Oranges CM, Sisti A, Sisti G. Labia minora reduction techniques: A comprehensive literature review. *Aesthet Surg J.* 2015;35:419–31.

17. Motakef S, Rodriguez-Feliz J, Chung MT, et al. Vaginal labiaplasty: Current practices and a simplified classification system for labial protrusion *Plast Reconstr Surg.* 2015;135: 774–88.

Clinical Evidence of the Effects of Female Genital Cosmetic Surgery

Lina Michala

Introduction

Female genital cosmetic surgery (FGCS) is advertised widely. The rise in uptake of FGCS [1] is paralleled by the rise in medical publications (Chapter 4 by Rodriguez, this volume). A PubMed search on labiaplasty suggests that the number of articles has tripled over the past few years, from 30 publications between 2008 and 2012 and a further 101 publications from 2013 to 2017 (Figure 6.1). However, high-quality studies that offer reliable evidence for such operations, particularly with regards to risks, benefits and long-term outcome, remain scarce. The vast majority of published peer-reviewed reports are small retrospective case reviews, in which patients are followed up for brief periods only and without the inclusion of a no-surgery or alternative treatment group for comparison. Most of the articles are published by the surgeons who are reporting on the results of operations they themselves have performed. In this chapter, I will review the available scientific evidence for labiaplasty and other FGCS procedures, focusing primarily on satisfaction post-surgery and risks of FGCS, especially

labiaplasty. I will furthermore outline the benchmarks for good science to which future clinical research in FGCS should aspire.

The 'Normal' Vulva

What is positioned (or sold) as 'normal' for vulval appearance and function transcends anatomical measurements (Chapter 3 by Braun, this volume). As surgeons, however, anatomy is where we must all begin. This is the first hurdle. Descriptions in anatomy or gynaecology textbooks are at best partial [2] (Chapter 2 by Crouch, this volume). This information has not been developed, for example, by studies that examine the variations in structure and appearance of female genitalia [3]. Aspects of the vagina remain entirely uncharted, not least the existence of the so-called G spot, and if it does exist, where it is located. Equally little has been written or known about the changes during adolescence, nor is there a staging of pubertal development for labial size and form similar to the Tanner staging for breast or pubic hair development. Parents and daughters who come forward

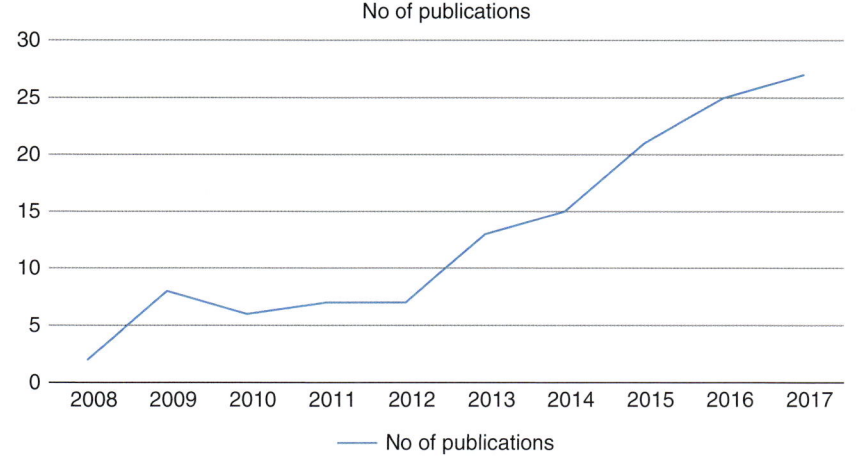

Figure 6.1 Number of publications on labiaplasty, 2008 to 2017.

with genital appearance concerns may both have been misled by traditional sex education (Chapter 11 by Lundberg, this volume). They rely on paediatricians and general practitioners who may not be in a position to guide them towards a more realistic and sympathetic understanding of their body [4]. All parties are potentially influenced by shared cultural biases.

Implied in most scientific publications aimed at medical professionals or lay people is that there is a standard prototype for female genitalia and it remains static throughout life. This assumption is reproduced in educational materials decade after decade. Myths have morphed into facts that have morphed into common sense, so that few women learn to expect that their genitals can be quite different from each other's and are, as for the rest of their body, transitional. The variations and usual changes across the lifespan, such as during pregnancy or following a vaginal delivery or menopause, are normal and nothing to fear. Girls and women who undergo FGCS procedures may not realise that the results, even if they were to match expectations exactly, are impermanent, because the body is not a static entity.

Guidelines from Scientific Bodies

In response to the increased demand for FGCS, a number of professional bodies have attempted to provide a framework for medical doctors to work within [5–11], but these are not professional standards that doctors have to adhere to. To put this into perspective, clinical recommendations in evidence-based health care should ideally be established on cumulative evidence leading to at least one randomised controlled trial. This would constitute what clinicians consider Level 1 evidence that makes its way to a Grade A recommendation. In the case of FGCS, guidance provided by professional bodies is at best Grade C recommendations, based usually on non-controlled studies and opinions.

The Society of Obstetricians and Gynaecologists of Canada states that terms such as vaginal rejuvenation, clitoral resurfacing and G-spot enhancement should be recognised as marketing terms only and that misleading advertisements are unethical [11]. In the relevant committee opinion paper, the American College of Obstetricians and Gynaecologists names these procedures 'not medically indicated' and stresses that their safety and effectiveness are not documented [7] (Table 6.1).

Scientific Evidence on Immediate Results and Patient Satisfaction

Labiaplasty is the most widely performed FGCS procedure. Scientific publications start to appear in the early 1970s [12]. From then and up to the late 1990s, only a handful of case reports or small case series (including up to four patients) can be identified. These reported on satisfaction on anecdotal grounds. From 2000 onwards, publications including larger numbers of women appeared in the literature with a better defined aim to report on postoperative patient satisfaction. However, most reports were still based on relatively small numbers of patients while larger series were flawed by a short follow-up and ad hoc evaluation of patient satisfaction, such as the operating surgeon asking patients face to face or on the telephone yes/no questions that were important from the surgeons' perspectives.

One of the first case series to comment on satisfaction and complications following labiaplasty was published in 2000 by Rouzier et al. [13], who reported on 163 patients with an age range from adolescence to menopause. This group assessed patients 1 month after labiaplasty with a simple questionnaire devised by the team and reported that 83% of patients were satisfied and only 4% declared that they would not undergo the procedure, given a second chance. In 2002 Pardo et al. [14] followed up 55 girls and women 2 months after surgery. The patients were assessed by a questionnaire devised by the researchers, who reported high satisfaction rates. In a similar fashion, Alter in 2008 [15], Cao et al. in 2012 [16], Gress in 2013 [17] and Gonzalez et al. in 2013 [18] reported on the satisfactory results of different labioplasty procedures performed in their departments. Although the series were fairly large, ranging from 50 to more than 800 patients, follow-up periods were short and the assessment of patients was non-standardised.

As early as the early 1990s some authors attempted to classify 'labial hypertrophy' in categories, and this classification has been used subsequently to offer a different surgical approach according to the degree of 'deformity'. Ellsworth et al. [19] used the Franco classification to determine whether de-epithelisation or edge or wedge resection should be performed. Based on the results of 12 patients, the authors designed an algorithm for triaging women to a specific type of operation. Later reviews of the literature [20, 21] further promoted the notion of

Table 6.1 Professional guidance on FGCS

Scientific Body	Type of Paper	Title	Year of Publication	Summary of Recommendations			
				Anatomy	Psychology	Advertising/Financial Conflicts	Complications
Society of Obstetricians and Gynaecologists of Canada	Policy Statement	Female Genital Cosmetic Surgery	2013	Help women understand anatomy and respect individual variations.	Ascertain the absence of major sexual or psychological dysfunction. Refer for assessment if identified.	Conflicts of interest when advertised. Advertising of FGCS is considered unethical.	Counsel on possible unintended consequences of cosmetic surgery to the genital area.
Royal College of Obstetricians and Gynaecologists	Ethical Opinion Paper	Ethical Considerations in Relation to Female Genital Cosmetic Surgery	2013	Provide accurate information about normal variations in female genitalia.	Offer counseling and other psychological treatments for body image distress.	Questions advertising practices. Reiterates General Medical Council and Advertising Standards Authority Guidance: publish factual information, encourage honest and trustworthy communication.	Irreversibility of labiaplasty. Inform about risks. Provide accurate written information sheet.
The Royal Australian and New Zealand College of Obstetricians and Gynaecologists	Statement	Vaginal 'Rejuvenation', Laser Ablation for Benign Conditions and Cosmetic Vaginal Procedures	2008, Amended 2016	Educate women on variations in appearance of external genitalia and normal physiological changes over time.	Recommends sexual counseling. Concerns on exploitation of vulnerable women.	Caution in accepting financial incentives from manufacturers of commercial products.	Discuss in detail. Scarring, adhesions, permanent disfigurement, infection, dyspareunia, altered sexual sensation.
The Royal Australian College of General Practitioners	Guidance	Female Genital Cosmetic Surgery: A Resource for General Practitioners and Other Health Professionals	2015	Use diagrams to educate the patient on normal female external genitalia anatomy; focus on sensorineural and functional aspects.	Take a psychosexual history, consider mental health and relationship or sexual abuse issues and refer accordingly.	Refers to Australian media code of conduct on body image, to place greater emphasis on diversity, positive body image and a focus on health rather than on body shape.	Potential risks associated with FGCS include bleeding, wound dehiscence, infection, scarring, sensorineural complications, dyspareunia, tearing of scar during childbirth, reduced lubrication.
American College of Obstetricians and Gynecologists, Committee on Gynecologic Practice	Committee Opinion	Vaginal 'Rejuvenation' and Cosmetic Vaginal Procedures	2007, Reaffirmed 2017	Engage in frank discussion with women regarding wide range of normal genitalia.	Evaluate for sexual dysfunction, explore non-surgical interventions, counselling.	Ethical concerns regarding marketing and franchising.	Inform regarding complications: infection, altered sensation, dyspareunia, adhesions and scarring.
American College of Obstetricians and Gynecologists, Committee on Adolescent Health Care	Committee Opinion	Breast and Labial Surgery in Adolescents	2017	Essential to have special knowledge of normal physical and psychosocial growth and development during adolescence.	Screen for body dysmorphic disorder.		Serious complications can occur (pain, painful scarring, dyspareunia, hematoma, edema and infection).
Swiss Society of Gynecology and Obstetrics	Letter of experts	Intervention Vulvo-vaginales sans Indications Medicale	2011	Inform women of individual variations in female external genitalia and changes during life.	Gynaecologists should address psychological concerns in women requesting FGCS.	Cosmetic indications only for FGCS. Caution to avoid fraud against medical insurance.	Document counselling of women regarding risks.

a specific technique application depending on labial size and form.

A study by Goodman et al. [22] attempted to offer a multicentre study of the effects of labiaplasty, vaginal rejuvenation and clitoral hood reduction, alone or in combination. Although the study involved 10 US centres and clarified surgical outcomes from different operators, only 258 out of 473 (55%) eligible patients answered the self-designed survey. A 91.6% satisfaction rate was mentioned. Although an overall significant improvement in sexual function was reported, on looking more closely at the results, 150 out of 237 patients who had undergone a surgical procedure reported either a negative (6 women) or no effect (144 women) as far as sexual satisfaction was concerned.

Veale et al. [23] published a prospective case-comparison study looking specifically at psychosexual outcomes using the Genital Appearance Satisfaction scale (GAS), the Hospital Anxiety and Depression Scale (HADS), the Pelvic Organ Prolapse-Urinary Incontinence Sexual Function Questionnaire (PISQ), the Body Image Quality of Life Inventory (BIQLI) and the Cosmetic Procedures Scale-Labia (COPS-L) that screens for body dysmorphic disorder. The researchers assessed women preoperatively and 3 months post-surgery and reported a significant improvement in genital appearance satisfaction that was maintained during a longer term follow-up. There was also significant improvement in the PISQ, COPS L and HADS anxiety scores, suggesting improved sexual function, relief from body dysmorphic disorder and decreased anxiety, respectively. However, the number of patients in the study was small, with 49 women participating out of 112 potential recruits (44%). Furthermore, the drop-out rate was high, with only just over half of the participating patients remaining in the study at the 3-month follow-up.

Subsequently, Goodman et al. [24] used a set of validated questionnaires to evaluate body image, genital self-image, sexual satisfaction and body esteem prospectively. The number of patients participating was 120. The authors included a control group of 50 women not desiring a labiaplasty. Patients were recruited consecutively and the participation rate was high, as was initial follow-up for body image and genital image. The authors reported a significant improvement for all of the variables assessed, including sexual satisfaction. However, on looking at results more closely, only 65 women completed the sexual satisfaction questionnaire and of these just over a third participated in the 2-year follow-up. The report omitted the number of women contacted for the research and, without knowing the participation rate, it is not possible to determine how generalisable the results area. Although the abstract states that sexual satisfaction values for the operated women 'surpassed' control values at 2 years post-surgery, this represents an over-conclusion given the flaws of the study.

More recently, a different type of study by Placik and Arkins [25] attempted to evaluate genital sensitivity after labia minora and clitoral hood reduction. The authors measured sensitivity to pressure using Semmes–Weinstein monofilaments, at five genital locations at baseline and at 3, 6 and 12 months after surgery. They reported a slight drop in pressure threshold at the edge of the labia that reached statistical significance, suggesting improved labial sensitivity at the point of excision. However only 37 out of a potential 120 women participated in the study, making it difficult to determine the generalisability of the results.

A positive improvement in providing evidence regarding labiaplasty is the involvement of psychologists in the independent evaluation of patients. In two recent studies by Sharp et al. [26, 27], patients were assessed, either through questionnaires or interviews, regarding their current satisfaction with a procedure performed in the recent past and whether they acknowledge an improvement, with regards to their previous state of sexual satisfaction or genital appearance satisfaction. Both studies reported improved outcomes after surgery, albeit decreasing, as follow-up time progressed. Interestingly, one in three patients retained their sexual difficulties after surgery. Once more, limitations stemmed from the small number of participants and the retrospective nature of the studies.

Evidence on results of FGCS procedures marketed as G-spot amplification or revirgination does not exist and therefore no scientific comment can be made on their effectiveness. However, a number of papers have recently been published on vaginal rejuvenation, aimed primarily at treating 'vaginal laxity'. Traditionally, vaginal laxity is treated surgically through colporrhaphy and perineoplasty, which are operations to tighten the vagina. Few studies exist to assess the effectiveness of surgical vaginal rejuvenation, and long-term follow-up beyond 6 months is non-existent. Pardo et al. looked at post-surgical results at 6 months in 53 women who underwent a colporrhaphy to treat vaginal laxity. Sexual function was assessed arbitrarily and was reported as improved in 90% of patients [28]. A later study in which a validated questionnaire was used to measure sexual function postoperatively found that vaginal tightness was achieved at the expense of dyspareunia (pain during sex), thus defeating the purpose of improving sexual function [29]. Recently, an American group assessed 78 women presenting with vaginal laxity post vaginal rejuvenation, using the Pelvic Organ Prolapse/Urinary Incontinence Sexual Questionnaire-12 (PISQ-12). The main drawback of the study was the vague definition of vaginal laxity, particularly as some women were as young as 25 years of age. The authors suggested improved postoperative sexual function scores in most domains of the PISQ, except for pain scores, which remained unchanged [30].

Newer non-surgical vaginal rejuvenation techniques, using radio frequency [31], laser [32] or silicone threads [33], aim to improve sexual function while avoiding invasive surgery. All techniques are relatively new, and evidence regarding results is again scanty. Radio frequency vaginal rejuvenation has been assessed in a well-designed multicentre randomised trial with a placebo arm (sham treatment), to assess improvement of vaginal laxity at 6 months after treatment [34]. In the treatment group, 43.5% of women had an improvement in vaginal laxity with improved FSFI scores. However, there was an unexpectedly high improvement, of 20%, in the placebo-treated group, who were blinded to the fact they were not receiving treatment, suggesting a strong placebo effect. The study was sponsored by the company marketing the radio frequency vaginal rejuvenation device. As vaginal rejuvenation is extremely profitable, more such studies are likely to be published in the future but the quality of the research should be even more closely scrutinised.

Reports of Side Effects and Evidence Regarding Risks

Labiaplasty entails edge excision, wedge resection or de-epithelialisation of a central part of the labium [19, 35] (Chapter 5 by Kavouni, this volume). It is usually performed as a day case under local or general anaesthetic. Although most labiaplasties are straightforward in technical terms, a number of complications have been reported, occurring mostly in the immediate postoperative period and some leading to revision surgery [20, 36]. Looking at the literature, it is difficult to reach robust conclusions about the actual risks. In a review of trends among American plastic surgeons published in 2012 [37], approximately one-tenth reported having reoperated for complications. Reasons leading to reoperation were dehiscence (wound separation) and poor healing, haematoma formation, infection or fistula. A proportion of surgeons reported reoperating as a result of inadequate initial resection, i.e., not removing enough labial tissue. Case series published over the past 15 years have reported minor self-resolving complications rates, such as poor healing and haematoma, in up to 40% of women, particularly with certain techniques, such as those in which de-epithelialisation of the middle section of the labium is performed [19, 38, 39]. Wound dehiscence was also commonly reported; however, in larger series, it reached at most a 6% rate [15–17]. No study collected information prospectively on complications, nor were complications the primary outcome of any retrospective study.

While vaginal rejuvenation appears to be a low-risk procedure in the short term, there are potential concerns regarding long-term effects, particularly as laser or radio frequency procedures can lead to tissue damage, which may lead to contractures and dyspareunia. Furthermore, there is a concern that energy may be diffused and affect adjacent organs, such as the rectum, urethra or the bladder [40, 41].

Future Research

Although there is a rise in the number of studies published, most represent a replication of previous publications, albeit with larger numbers and using psychometric scales. The methodology may appear more credible but the newer studies have not improved the quality of the evidence. For example, no study has included two groups of women with comparable labial dimensions, with one group undergoing labiaplasty and another not. Another method would be to compare equally dissatisfied women who choose FGCS or a psychological intervention (Chapter 13 by Brotto, Bryce and Todd, this volume). It is important to assess pre- and post-intervention along anatomical, psychological and sexual parameters and to repeat the assessments up to 3 years post-intervention. Response rates should always be included in any report and, in order to reduce bias, the data should be analysed by blinded independent researchers.

In addition, little is known at this current time on how a previous FGCS will affect childbirth. Will there be a higher incidence of perineal tears, for example? Also, how will pregnancy or labour and delivery affect the result of a previous FGCS? Another area to consider is whether healing following a FGCS is affected by race, type of skin or susceptibility to keloid scarring.

Given the social pressure, vulval appearance dissatisfaction may affect many more women than the subgroup who progress to surgery and even repeat operations. There is a paucity of studies that investigate the factors that underpin vulval appearance dissatisfaction/distress and those that underpin progression to surgery and post-surgical dis/satisfaction. This kind of research can help us to understand the differences between women and develop a wider range of responses. It is only through knowing what FGCS is for that we can define and measure outcomes clearly. Only then is it possible to arrive at Grades A and B recommendations. Women deserve to be able to base their decisions on good science.

Conclusion

Data on success rates and complications of labiaplasty and other cosmetic genital procedures are scanty. The past 5 years have seen an attempt to better assess women who undergo FGCS, at least for research purposes. A few recent studies include an independent investigator rather than the actual FGCS operator, and try to assess patients more objectively, including comparison with a control group. A step forward is the use of validated questionnaires, addressing satisfaction with genital appearance following the procedure and its effects on sexual function. However, selection bias still remains, as only a small proportion of patients undergoing labiaplasties are included in studies, and a high drop-out rate means that long-term follow-up will not be easily available.

Potential suggestions for research in the future would be to randomise patients, in order to objectively correlate the effect of surgery to their quality of life and sexuality. Results of FGCS have not been tested over time, and what remains to be determined is how genital appearance and function can be affected by pregnancy, childbirth or menopausal changes in women who have previously undergone

an FGCS and how the FGCS itself may interfere with the changes expected to occur during these normal transitions.

References

1. Lowenstein L, Salonia A, Shechter A, Porst H, Burri A, Reisman Y. Physicians' attitude toward female genital plastic surgery: A multinational survey. *J Sex Med.* 2014;11(1):33–9.

2. Andrikopoulou M, Michala L, Creighton SM, Liao LM. The normal vulva in medical textbooks. *J Obstet Gynaecol.* 2013;33(7):648–50.

3. Lloyd J, Crouch NS, Minto CL, Liao LM, Creighton SM. Female genital appearance: "normality" unfolds. *BJOG.* 2005;112(5):643–6.

4. Michala L, Koliantzaki S, Antsaklis A. Protruding labia minora: Abnormal or just uncool? *J Psychosom Obstet Gynaecol.* 2011;32(3):154–6.

5. Committee on Gynecologic Practice, American College of Obstetricians and Gynecologists. Committee Opinion No. 686: Breast and labial surgery in adolescents. *Obstet Gynecol.* 2017;129(1): e17–e19.

6. Wyss P, Pok J, Hagmann P, et al. Interventions vulvo-vaginales sans indication medicale. Lettre d'experts No. 39. Societe Suisse de Gynecologie et d'Obstetrique; 2011.

7. Committee on Gynecologic Practice, American College of Obstetricians and Gynecologists. ACOG Committee Opinion No. 378: Vaginal "rejuvenation" and cosmetic vaginal procedures. *Obstet Gynecol.* 2007;110(3):737–8.

8. RCOG Ethics Committee, Ethical considerations in relation to female genital cosmetic surgery (FGCS), RCOG, October 2013.

9. The Royal Australian and New Zealand College of Obstetricians and Gynaecologists. Vaginal 'rejuvenation, laser ablation for benign conditions and cosmetic vaginal procedures. RANZCOG, March 2015.

10. The Royal Australian College of General Practitioners. Female genital cosmetic surgery. A resource for general practitioners and other health professionals. RACGP, July 2015.

11. Shaw D, Lefebvre G, Bouchard C, et al. Female genital cosmetic surgery. *J Obstet Gynaecol Can.* 2013;35(12): 1108–12.

12. Capraro VJ. Congenital anomalies. *Clin Obstet Gynecol.* 1971;14(4):988–1012.

13. Rouzier R, Louis-Sylvestre C, Paniel BJ, Haddad B. Hypertrophy of labia minora: Experience with 163 reductions. *Am J Obstet Gynecol.* 2000;182(1 Pt 1):35–40.

14. Pardo J, Sola V, Ricci P, Guilloff E. Laser labioplasty of labia minora. *Int J Gynaecol Obstet.* 2006;93(1):38–43.

15. Alter GJ. Aesthetic labia minora and clitoral hood reduction using extended central wedge resection. *Plast Reconstr Surg.* 2008;122(6):1780–9.

16. Cao YJ, Li FY, Li SK, et al. A modified method of labia minora reduction: The de-epithelialised reduction of the central and posterior labia minora. *J Plast Reconstr Aesthet Surg.* 2012;65(8):1096–102.

17. Gress S. Composite reduction labiaplasty. *Aesthetic Plast Surg.* 2013;37(4):674–83.

18. Gonzalez F, Dass D, Almeida B. Custom flask labiaplasty. *Ann Plast Surg.* 2015;75(3):266–71.

19. Ellsworth WA, Rizvi M, Lypka M, et al. Techniques for labia minora reduction: An algorithmic approach. *Aesthetic Plast Surg.* 2010 34(1):105–10.

20. Oranges CM, Sisti A, Sisti G. Labia minora reduction techniques: A comprehensive literature review. *Aesthet Surg J.* 2015;35(4):419–31.

21. Motakef S, Rodriguez-Feliz J, Chung MT, Ingargiola MJ, Wong VW, Patel A. Vaginal labiaplasty: Current practices and a simplified classification system for labial protrusion. *Plast Reconstr Surg.* 2015;135(3):774–88.

22. Goodman MP, Placik OJ, Benson RH, III, et al. A large multicenter outcome study of female genital plastic surgery. *J Sex Med.* 2010;7(4 Pt 1):1565–77.

23. Veale D, Naismith I, Eshkevari E, et al. Psychosexual outcome after labiaplasty: A prospective case-comparison study. *Int Urogynecol J.* 2014;25(6):831–9.

24. Goodman MP, Placik OJ, Matlock DL, et al. Evaluation of body image and sexual satisfaction in women undergoing female genital plastic/cosmetic surgery. *Aesthet Surg J.* 2016;36(9):1048–57.

25. Placik OJ, Arkins JP. A prospective evaluation of female external genitalia sensitivity to pressure following labia minora reduction and clitoral hood reduction. *Plast Reconstr Surg.* 2015;136(4):442e–452e.

26. Sharp G, Tiggemann M, Mattiske J. Psychological outcomes of labiaplasty: A prospective study. *Plast Reconstr Surg.* 2016;138(6):1202–9.

27. Sharp G, Mattiske J, Vale KI. Motivations, expectations, and experiences of labiaplasty: A qualitative study. *Aesthet Surg J.* 2016;36(8):920–8.

28. Pardo JS, Urmanche A, Wilman S, Wiener J. Phonetic convergence across multiple measures and model talkers. *Atten Percept Psychophys.* 2017;79(2):637–59.

29. Abedi P, Jamali S, Tadayon M, Parhizkar S, Mogharab F. Effectiveness of selective vaginal tightening on sexual function among reproductive aged women in Iran with vaginal laxity: A quasi-experimental study. *J Obstet Gynaecol Res.* 2014; 40(2):526–31.

30. Moore RD, Miklos JR, Chinthakanan O. Evaluation of sexual function outcomes in women undergoing vaginal rejuvenation/vaginoplasty procedures for symptoms of vaginal laxity/decreased vaginal sensation utilizing validated sexual function questionnaire (PISQ-12). *Surg Technol Int.* 2014;24:253–60.

31. Millheiser LS, Pauls RN, Herbst SJ, Chen BH. Radiofrequency treatment of vaginal laxity after vaginal delivery: Nonsurgical vaginal tightening. *J Sex Med.* 2010;7(9):3088–95.

32. Filippini M, Del DE, Negosanti F, et al. Fractional CO_2 laser: From skin rejuvenation to vulvo-vaginal reshaping. *Photomed Laser Surg.* 2017;35(3):171–5.

33. Park TH, Park HJ, Whang KW. Functional vaginal rejuvenation with elastic silicone threads: A 4-year experience with 180 patients. *J Plast Surg Hand Surg.* 2015; 49(1):36–9.

34. Krychman M, Rowan CG, Allan BB, et al. Effect of single-treatment, surface-cooled radiofrequency therapy on vaginal laxity and female sexual function: The VIVEVE I Randomized Controlled Trial. *J Sex Med.* 2017;14(2):215–25.

35. Dobbeleir JM, Landuyt KV, Monstrey SJ. Aesthetic surgery of the female genitalia. *Semin Plast Surg.* 2011;25(2):130–41.

36. Liao LM, Michala L, Creighton SM. Labial surgery for well women: A review of the literature. *BJOG.* 2010;117(1):20–5.

37. Mirzabeigi MN, Moore JH, Jr., Mericli AF, et al. Current trends in vaginal labioplasty: A survey of plastic surgeons. *Ann Plast Surg.* 2012;68(2):125–34.

38. Solanki NS, Tejero-Trujeque R, Stevens-King A, Malata CM. Aesthetic and functional reduction of the labia minora using the Maas and Hage technique. *J Plast Reconstr Aesthet Surg.* 2010;63(7):1181–5.

39. Giraldo F, Gonzalez C, de HF. Central wedge nymphectomy with a 90-degree Z-plasty for aesthetic reduction of the labia minora. *Plast Reconstr Surg.* 2004;113(6):1820–5.

40. Singh A, Swift S, Khullar V, Digesu GA. Laser vaginal rejuvenation: Not ready for prime time. *Int Urogynecol J.* 2015;26(2):163–4.

41. Barbara G, Facchin F, Buggio L, Alberico D, Frattaruolo MP, Kustermann A. Vaginal rejuvenation: Current perspectives. *Int J Womens Health.* 2017;9:513–19.

The Law and Ethics of Female Genital Cutting

Arianne Shahvisi and Brian D. Earp

Introduction

Nontherapeutic female genital cutting (FGC) typically conjures associations of gender oppression and child abuse in the Western imagination. More commonly described as 'female genital mutilation' or 'FGM', such cutting has been roundly condemned and legislated against [1]. Yet FGM/C is not exclusively a practice of the Other, as is often assumed. In Western countries, the demand for a range of surgical procedures collectively known as female genital cosmetic surgery (FGCS) is rising [2], as women – and, increasingly, teenage girls [3] – pursue a perceived aesthetic ideal identified with 'designer vaginas', including petite clitoral hoods, non-protruding labia, and pre-pubescent hairlessness, apparently modelled on exemplars from pornography [4]. Moreover, some forms of medically unnecessary cosmetic or 'normalising' surgery performed on intersex children before an age of consent – such as 'feminising' cliteroplasty to reduce the size of healthy, albeit larger than average clitorises [5] – are consistent with Western legal definitions of female genital mutilation, but are largely accepted and still regularly performed [6].

A word on terminology. As 'mutilation' is a value-laden term, indicating intentional disfigurement or damage, we consider that its use (a) fails to accurately reflect the motivations of communities within which the class of relevant practices is common (no loving parents seek to mutilate their child), and (b) tends to prefigure the debate, introducing moral biases that are not imposed on analogous forms of non-therapeutic genital cutting which are more familiar in Western contexts, such as FGCS or male circumcision (see Box 7.1), both of which are typically picked out by more neutral descriptors. We therefore favour the terms 'female genital cutting' (FGC), 'female genital cosmetic surgery' (FGCS) and, where applicable, 'male genital cutting' (MGC) or male circumcision, and we will use these terms throughout the chapter. Where it is necessary to use the term 'FGM', for

example, when referencing the activist/advocacy literature devoted to the elimination of such practices, it will appear in scare quotes to draw attention to its disfavoured status among scholars of genital cutting [7–9].

In the second section, we describe the different varieties of female genital cutting, focusing on the differences and commonalities between (a) purportedly 'mutilating' forms of FGC and (b) Western-style FGCS. The third section interrogates the law in the United Kingdom (and other Western contexts) in relation to each class of procedure. The fourth section highlights the inconsistencies arising from the differential legislative approaches, while the fifth section explores some of the problematic assumptions that underwrite these inconsistencies. The sixth section concludes.

Varieties of Genital Cutting

According to the World Health Organization (WHO), 'female genital mutilation' refers to any procedure "involving partial or total removal of the external female genitalia or other injury to the female genital organs for non-medical reasons" [10]. The term therefore covers a loose assemblage of different interventions, carried out by different groups for different reasons in different settings, ranging from a prick to the clitoral hood (which does not remove tissue and is thus less invasive than male circumcision; see Box 7.1) to the excision of the external clitoris followed by suturing of the vaginal opening (known as infibulation). These interventions may occur in a hospital setting or a rural village; they may be carried out by a medical practitioner or a medically untrained ritual provider; they may be performed with sterile instruments and anaesthesia or with a septic tool and no pain control whatsoever [34]. As noted, we will use 'female genital cutting' (FGC) to refer to all such non-therapeutic procedures – non-therapeutic in the sense that they are imposed on healthy genitalia and are not intended to treat

BOX 7.1 Comparison to Male Genital Cutting

Non-therapeutic male genital cutting (MGC) ranges from ritual pricking (e.g., *hatafat dam brit*), to piercing, scraping the inside of the urethra, bloodletting, shaft scarring and/or foreskin slitting (among, e.g., various ethnic groups in Papua New Guinea) [11], to circumcision as it is traditionally performed on male newborns in Judaism and generally in the United States (tearing of the membrane that fuses the immature foreskin to the head of the penis followed by excision of the majority of the foreskin) [12], to *metzitzah b'peh* (the same followed by direct oral suction of the wound, risking herpes infection, performed on more than 3,000 babies in New York City each year within the ultra-Orthodox Jewish community) [7], to non-sterilised, un-anaesthetised circumcisions performed in the bush during rites of passage in Eastern and Southern Africa [13], to highly traumatic mass cutting of pre-teen boys carried out on school tables in the Philippines (*tuli*) [14], to forced circumcision of men following political conflict in various countries [15], to subincision (slicing open the underside of the penis lengthwise, often through to the urethra) in Aboriginal Australia [16], to involuntary castration (now rare but occasionally documented among the *hijras* of India). The extent of cutting, tools used, skill of the practitioner, age of the initiate and so on vary widely across circumstances, leading to a heterogeneous risk profile both within and across types. There is also considerable variation in associated social and symbolic meanings (e.g., sealing a divine covenant, punishing an enemy, mimicking menstruation, proving oneself as a man, basis for marriageability, perceived hygiene, ritual purification, conformity to peer pressure, etc.) as well as physical context (e.g., sometimes medicalised, often not), depending on the group in question.

The most common form of MGC is circumcision. Male circumcision involves the partial or total removal of the foreskin of the penis – an elastic sleeve of erogenous tissue that normally covers and protects the glans – occasionally to address a medical problem, but most often for ethnoreligious or cultural reasons [17]. In Western countries the surgery is typically performed on healthy newborn babies or young male children as part of a medicalised birth custom, as in the United States [18], or in the context of a religious ritual, for example, among practicing Muslims and Jews. Such non-therapeutic circumcision of infant males is regarded as legal throughout the Global North, with few restrictions or exceptions [19].

Supporters of circumcision tend to view the procedure as relatively harmless – except in the case of 'botched' operations – possibly owing to a lack of awareness of the anatomical properties of the excised tissue (if the tissue itself has value, its sheer removal is a harm) [20]. Increasingly, men who were circumcised in infancy or early childhood, that is, before they were old enough to give or withhold their informed consent, are voicing distress and opposition to the surgery, often citing a lack of personal choice concerning an irreversible alteration to their most private sexual anatomy [21]. In addition to this perceived violation of their genital autonomy, there are also inherent (or highly probable) effects of early circumcision that some such men regard as deleterious. These include the presence of scar tissue and associated discoloration, inability to engage in sexual acts requiring foreskin motility [22], elimination of the parts of the penis most sensitive to light touch [23] and irritation and possible altered sensitivity of the glans.

Common side effects include meatal stenosis (pathological narrowing of the urethral opening) [24], bleeding, infections and incomplete skin removal requiring revision surgery. Additional side effects of unknown frequency include painful erections due to excessive skin removal, partial or complete amputation of the organ due to surgical error, urinary problems, fistulae, skin bridges and cysts [25]. Finally, death is a possible outcome: in the United States, early deaths following circumcision in clinical settings occur at a rate of approximately 1 for every 50,000 circumcisions [26]. In rural settings, such as among the Xhosa of South Africa, deaths as well as penile amputations are far more common: between 2008 and 2014, more than half a million Xhosa boys were hospitalised due to botched circumcisions in the Eastern Cape alone, while between 2006 and 2010 there were 269 recorded deaths among this group and 146 penile amputations [27, 28].

In settings where circumcision is relatively common, such as the United States, prophylactic health benefits are often cited in support of the practice [29]. However, the evidence is contested and is associated primarily with adult, voluntary circumcision in sub-Saharan Africa, not newborn circumcision in economically developed regions with advanced health care systems [30]. In any case, the claimed health benefits can be achieved non-surgically through, e.g., safe sex practices and basic hygiene. Accordingly, the vast majority of international health authorities to have issued formal statements on the health benefits and risks associated with newborn and early childhood male circumcision have concluded that the benefits do not outweigh the risks [31]. Even if they did, however, removing healthy tissue as prophylaxis without consent is not automatically morally acceptable. Consider that performing non-consensual mastectomies on adolescent girls with high-risk genetic profiles in order to guard against future breast cancer would not be tolerated. Similarly, neonatal labiaplasty, though it might conceivably reduce the risk of certain labial cancers or other such problems, is not seriously entertained as a means of health promotion [32]. Although prophylactic tonsillectomies were once common, they are no longer regularly performed; moreover, the tonsils, in contrast to the genitals, are not a visually prominent, psycho-sexually significant external organ. Among ethicists and legal scholars, it is now increasingly argued that male infants and young boys, just like female infants and young girls, have a strong moral interest in having their genital integrity preserved until they are old enough to make an informed, personal decision [33].

a recognised disease nor are required to preserve or restore functionality (sexual, reproductive, urinary or otherwise). In practice, FGC almost always involves the clinically unnecessary modification of vulvar tissue in order to adhere to perceived religious or cultural norms or ideals.

Table 7.1 shows the extent of the similarities between the set of practices described by the WHO as 'FGM' and those more commonly described as FGCS. As has been noted elsewhere [35], genital cutting procedures are diverse, falling on a wide spectrum of severity, in part because the motivations for the procedures – both conscious and unconscious, historical and contemporary – are likewise diverse. Some groups, for example, are openly committed to tempering the sexual desires of women, as is apparent in many contexts throughout Egypt, where clitoridectomy (partial or total removal of the external clitoris) is common [36]. In other contexts, the procedure marks a transition from childhood to adulthood and may have little to do with reducing sexual desire or exerting sexual control [37]. In still others, such as among the Muslim Malay population of southern Thailand, both boys and girls are subjected to genital cutting as a form of ritual purification as well as to symbolise full acceptance into the Islamic community. For their part, the boys have their foreskins removed in a public ceremony between the ages of 7 and 12, while the girls experience a 'prick' to the clitoral hood shortly after birth [38, 39]. Similar cutting occurs among the Dawoodi Bohra sect of Shia Islam, whose followers are concentrated in Gujarat, India, and Karachi, Pakistan: the boys are circumcised, and the girls – in the typical case – have part of their clitoral hood cut or removed in a practice known as *khatna*, with stated reasons for both kinds of cutting ranging from 'religious purposes' to 'physical hygiene and cleanliness' [40].

The WHO collects all such (female) practices together under the banner of 'FGM' [41]. Although some nuance is introduced through seemingly arbitrary divisions into types and sub-types, the WHO

typology is not able to ground a principled distinction between (typically African, Middle Eastern or Southeast Asian) so-called mutilations and (chiefly European and North American) so-called cosmetic genital procedures. In the second column of Table 7.1, we present a parallel typology of practices which are standard within FGCSs. The table is organised to exhibit the commonalities between the component practices.

Table 7.1 shows that for each component of the 'FGM' typology, there is a close analogue within the FGCS typology. Alterations of the clitoris, labia and vaginal opening are observed in both sets of practices, with considerable variation both between and across cases as to the degree of tissue damage or removal. Instead of using umbrella terms such as 'FGM' or FGCS, then, it is likely to be more illuminating in most cases to be specific. Thus, one should refer to (1) particular procedures (e.g., labiaplasty, cliteridectomy, hoodectomy, infibulation); (2) the extent of the procedure, along with the means by which it is carried out – i.e., with which instruments and how skilfully – and the associated risk/benefit profile (both medical and non-medical); and (3) the relevant context: physical, psychological and social/symbolic. As it stands, the terms 'FGM' and FGCS are proposed as stable categories not on the basis of the acts that actually fall within them, but instead by the perceived *reasons* for undertaking those acts (e.g., 'non-medical reasons', 'to oppress women' and so on).

That said, there are some differences between the two categories. The first is that the practices known as 'FGM' are generally not performed in a regulated medical setting (although they are increasingly being performed in medicalised settings in the communities in which they are common and customary) [54], while those within the FGCS typology are usually performed by trained professionals in medical or similar facilities (although there are growing concerns about a lack of regulation) [55].

A second potential difference concerns the age at which the cutting is typically performed – i.e., usually

Table 7.1 Comparing 'FGM' and FGCS

	'FGM'	FGCS
Procedures and typology	Type I: **Alterations of the clitoris**, within which type 1a is the partial or total removal of the clitoral hood, and type 1b is the partial or total removal of the clitoral hood and the (external portion of the)[a] clitoris.	**Alterations of the clitoris,** including clitoral reshaping [42], clitoral unhooding [43], and clitoridectomy or cliteroplasty [44] (also common in "intersex" surgeries) [5, 6].
	Type II: **Alterations of the labia**, within which type IIa is the partial or total removal of the labia minora, type IIb is the partial or total removal of the labia minora and/or the (external)[a] clitoris and type IIc is the partial or total removal of the labia minora, labia majora and (external)[a] clitoris.	**Alterations of the labia**, including trimming of the labia minora and/or majora, also known as 'labiaplasty' [42, 43].
	Type III: **Alterations of the vaginal opening**, within which type IIIa is the partial or total removal and appositioning of the labia minora, and type IIIb is the partial or total removal and appositioning of the labia majora, both as ways of narrowing the vaginal opening.	**Alterations of the vaginal opening,** typified by narrowing of the vaginal opening, variously known as 'vaginal tightening', 'vaginal rejuvenation' [45] or 'hymen repair' [46].
	Type IV: **Miscellaneous,** including piercing, pricking, scraping and cauterisation.	**Miscellaneous**, including piercing [47], tattooing [48] and liposuction [49].
Example high-prevalence geographies	Depending on the procedure: Somalia, Sierra Leone, Guinea, Djibouti, Egypt, Mali, Sudan, Senegal, Eritrea, Ethiopia, Mauritania, Liberia, Burkina Faso, Gambia, Guinea Bissau, Kenya, Nigeria, Chad, Cote d'Ivoire and concomitant diaspora communities [50].	North America, Australia, Europe [51].
Actor	Traditional practitioner, midwife, clinical worker or paramedic, surgeon.	Surgeon, tattoo artist, body piercer.
Age at which performed	Depending on the procedure/community: typically around puberty, but ranging from infancy to adulthood [32].	Typically in adulthood, but increasingly on adolescent girls [3]; intersex surgeries (e.g., cliteroplasty) more common in infancy, but ranging through adolescence and adulthood [52].
Legal status in the UK and similar regimes	Unlawful	Lawful

[a] The WHO wrongly equates the external portion of the clitoris (i.e., the part that protrudes outside the body) with the entire clitoris, thereby diminishing the anatomical and sexual significance of the latter. Most of the clitoris, including the majority of its erectile tissues and structures necessary for orgasm, is underneath the superficial skin layer of the body – like an iceberg – and therefore cannot be removed without major surgery (which does not occur in any recognised form of 'FGM'). This fact may explain why sexual pleasure and orgasm are reported at higher than expected rates in women who have experienced various forms of genital cutting [53].

minor girls for 'FGM', usually adult women for FGCS – but there is overlap here as well. First, in many African societies, female and male genital cutting ceremonies constitute the very ritual by which adult status is conferred in the community, which complicates the question of consent as well as adult/child designations [56]. Second, staying just within the USA, UK and other Western contexts, non-therapeutic genital cutting – e.g., cosmetic labiaplasty – is increasingly performed on female children and adolescents well before the age of legal majority [57].

The final difference is their status in law: in Western countries FGM of any type is illegal (in the UK and Australia, this is true regardless of the age at which it is performed), while in these same countries, FGCS is treated as legal despite technically meeting the same criteria [58].

The Status of the Law

In this chapter, we take UK law as a case study. However, similar laws apply throughout the Western world [59], where increased migration of FGC-prevalent communities, coupled with a growing focus on FGC as a contested site of political attention, have led to pressure to address FGC either in dedicated legislation, or under existing laws.

In England, Wales and Northern Ireland, the FGM Act 2003 holds that "to excise, infibulate, or otherwise mutilate any part of a girl's labia minora, majora or clitoris" is an offense with a maximum sentence of fourteen years [60]. The legislation has two puzzling features. First, it stipulates that "Girl includes woman" and therefore equates the consent capacities of adult women to those of children. Second, the legislation contains a caveat to permit genital alterations where they are deemed necessary to the "mental health" of a person, while noting that it is "immaterial" for purpose of making such assessments whether the person requesting the alteration "or any other person believes that the operation is required as a matter of custom or ritual."

These rather confusing qualifications were evidently inserted to ring-fence access to FGCS, by portraying such procedures as necessary to the mental health of some women (as judged by their cosmetic surgeons), while preventing 'traditional' FGC, which is more readily interpreted as being performed for reasons that qualify as customary or ritualistic, from slipping through under the mental health clause. Dustin [61] suggests that the cosmetic surgery lobby may have played a key role in securing the future of FGCS when the legislation was being drafted.

Yet one could argue that FGCS also qualifies as being motivated by custom or ritual. As noted by Crouch and colleagues, it is "difficult to see how FGCS could be anything other than cultural" [62]. For as Edwards argues, "any woman's choice to have a procedure on her genitals cannot be separated from the culture in which this decision is made" [63]. Highly restrictive aesthetic ideals, widespread anatomical ignorance about the range of 'normal' appearances for the vulva, marketing campaigns designed to prey on bodily insecurities and normatively questionable social pressures undoubtedly threaten 'mental health' and thus play a role in motivating requests for FGCS [64]. In short, "the rationale [for cutting] cannot be separated from cultural associations" regardless of the culture in which it occurs [63].

Similarly, it is plausible that there may be potentially severe adverse consequences to the mental health of a person who is denied FGC if she lives within an FGC-prevalent community, identifies with the practice, regards modified vulvae as normal or beautiful (or unmodified vulvae as abnormal or ugly) [7, 9, 56, 86] and so on. But if, as it seems reasonable to argue, problematic cultural norms or expectations are ultimately to blame for any such psychological anguish – such that the norms and expectations, rather than female bodies, should be

changed [46] – they are certainly no less to blame for women's 'mental health' issues in the majority culture, which are used to justify FGCS.

Perhaps the difference in law can be grounded in the fact that FGCS is medically safer than FGC. One might indeed contend that the first is safer under current legislation, as it is usually performed in clinical contexts, while the latter must be performed 'underground' in Western countries because it is unlawful. Yet the division is not so tidy. First, in communities where FGC is common, the cutting is often performed in medical settings prior to immigration: according to the WHO, in some FGC-prevalent countries, "one-third or more of women had their daughter subjected to the practice by a trained health professional" [10]. By contrast, Western-style 'cosmetic' genital piercing, a legal form of FGCS, typically takes place in a non-clinical environment such as a tattoo parlour and is only minimally regulated [55].

Moreover, depending on the type of cutting, medical training does not guarantee superior skill: for example, in some communities, FGC – similar to MGC performed by a Jewish *mohel* – is carried out by a highly experienced circumciser for whom the cutting is her primary occupation. Thus, medicalisation per se does not eliminate, nor even necessarily reduce, the risk of complications, as the WHO also notes [10] (but see [65]).

Accordingly, many of the complications and risks are similar for FGC and FGCS where the type (as indicated in Table 7.1) matches. Even where FGCS of various types are performed by a licensed surgeon, the following complications are commonly noted: infection, healing problems, adhesion, dyspareunia, bleeding and effects on sexual pleasure [66]. These are strongly redolent of the sorts of complications that are often described as following from many instances of FGC, though of course, non-clinical environments and instruments, where applicable, may render these complications more likely and more severe [67].

Finally, as noted earlier, the presumed difference between FGC and FGCS in terms of the age at which the cutting takes place is not sufficient to ground such divergent laws: some FGC procedures, such as re-infibulation, are requested by adult women [68], while some FGCS procedures are performed on adolescent girls. Nevertheless, in all Western contexts, 'FGM' is unlawful, while FGCS procedures are presumed to be lawful. The 'mental health' caveat within UK law in particular exemplifies the difficulty in outlawing one set of procedures while protecting access to a set of procedures that is identical or nearly identical in physical terms. The difference, in the eyes of the law, then seems to rest on certain stereotypes concerning the *reason* for which the procedure is undertaken, a matter we will take up in the following sections.

Interrogating Inconsistencies

All three of FGCS, FGC and MGC involve the non-therapeutic modification or removal of healthy, erotogenic tissue. While there is a lively debate about the average (net) effects of these practices on health [29, 30, 31, 69] and sexual pleasure [22, 30, 70, 86], what is often lost in such discussions is that no one is an embodied statistical average: genital cutting affects different individuals differently, depending on the type and extent of cutting, whether and what kind of pain control is used, the age at which it is performed, the skill of the practitioner, one's mind-set going into the cutting – or later reflecting on it or its effects – and so on [71]. Given such vast individual differences, arguably the more pressing question for ethicists working within a Western medico-legal context is whether the person in question can consent to the procedure and thereby exercise bodily autonomy, often characterised as a (human) right [72].

As noted, the capacity of adult women to *choose* FGC or FGCS is sometimes disputed, often along racial lines, a discussion to which we will return later. But the question of consent is perhaps most salient in the case of children. Supporters of childhood genital cutting note that infants and young children are pre-autonomous and therefore incapable of either giving or withholding their informed consent, not only to genital cutting, but to any significant parental action that affects them [73]. Therefore, they suggest, it is up to the parents to decide whether to cut the child's genitals. But such cutting is typically irreversible: depriving a child of the opportunity to remain genitally intact is also to deprive the eventual adult of the same opportunity. Plainly, a child's temporary lack of capacity to make certain informed, mature decisions about the state or condition of their own body does not create a 'blank cheque' for parents to authorise whatever permanent body alterations they may choose [74].

Granting this point, some authors argue that the permissibility of a given act of childhood genital cutting – usually presumed to fall somewhere beneath an arbitrary and unspecified threshold of harm [75] – depends on the *reason* for its performance, that is, the conscious or unconscious motive(s) of the parents or wider community [73]. Some motives, at least for certain kinds of non-therapeutic childhood genital cutting, appear to be regarded as acceptable in Western societies, while other motives are regarded as unacceptable.

For example, discussants who oppose even less physically invasive forms of FGC carried out prior to an age of consent (for example, ritual nicking), while at the same time tolerating or even advocating more physically invasive forms of MGC carried out prior to an age of consent (chiefly, infant male circumcision), tend to base their arguments on the premise that male circumcision is a religious requirement, at least for some groups, while FGC is not. The argument then proceeds to claim that if there is a 'religious' motive for childhood genital cutting, then the cutting can be justified, whether morally or legally.

However, the premise is false, so the argument is unsound. First, FGC is very often regarded by its supporters as an explicitly Islamic practice with the same or similar scriptural standing as male circumcision [7, 65]. While it is true that FGC, like MGC, is not mentioned in Koranic scripture, both are noted in the Hadith, a record of the teachings of the Prophet Mohammed. On this basis, some Muslim authorities argue that FGC is in fact obligatory (though this view is far from universal) [76]. Certainly, in Judaism and Christianity, it is widely held that 'binding' religious obligations can stem from extra-biblical sources, such as rabbinic commentaries or papal encyclicals: the notion that a practice can only be 'religious' if it is grounded in a literal reading of a group's primary scripture is absurd [65].

Second, male circumcision is often performed for merely 'cultural', rather than specifically religious, reasons, and yet it is broadly tolerated even in those cases. Christians in Africa, for instance, often practise infant male circumcision not because they view it as an explicit requirement of their own religion, but rather because the practice is widespread in the communities alongside which they live [77]. In the United States, circumcision of newborn boys is performed mostly in accordance with perceived social and aesthetic norms by those who place no religious stake in the surgery whatsoever, with statements such as "the boy should look like his father" held up as common explanations [18, 78]. Even many Jews who circumcise are atheists or otherwise non-religious, yet choose to continue the tradition for various reasons including a sense of shared history or ethnic identity [79]. In a similar vein, a study in Australia showed that three times as many parents opted to have their newborn son circumcised to continue a 'family tradition' than to fulfil a perceived religious obligation [80].

This leads to a dilemma. If male circumcision should be permitted generally and for any reason because in *some* groups it is regarded as an explicitly religious practice, then relatively more mild forms of FGC that are regarded by *some* groups as religiously required should be given equal consideration, and should also be tolerated for all groups regardless of the reason. Indeed, some prominent defenders of ritual male circumcision, aware of the existing double standard (see Box 7.1), have recently begun to argue that 'mild' forms of FGC should in fact be tolerated in Western law, presumably to ensure that the legal status of male circumcision remains unquestioned [65, 81]. Alternatively, one might argue that male circumcision should be permitted only when it is done for explicitly religious reasons (which would exclude most US American circumcisions, and might also exclude non-religious Jewish and Islamic circumcisions that would otherwise be done for merely 'cultural' reasons), in which case, by analogy, only groups that regard FGC as religiously required would be permitted to perform the cutting, and all others disallowed. Finally, one could argue that *neither* male nor female non-therapeutic childhood genital cutting should be permitted,

regardless of the religious motives of the parents [82].

Whichever option one favours, the common emphasis in this discourse on 'religion' versus 'culture' is telling. The apparent assumption is that religious norms are categorically different from, and more important than, 'merely' cultural norms. However, it is not obvious that there is a firm line – whether in practice or conceptually – between what is religious and what is cultural [77], nor is it obvious that one should be elevated above the other as 'legitimate' grounds for cutting the genitals of a child [83].

Even more peculiar, the false dichotomy is inconsistently applied. For example, it is often argued that (adult) FGCS is more acceptable than (adult) FGC because the former are *not* motivated by a strong cultural imperative [85]. That is, FGCS is presented as a procedure which is *chosen* by those who request it, which makes it at least plausibly permissible, whereas FGC is presented as an *obligation* for those who request it (by virtue of being a ritual or custom), which then renders it impermissible because it is presumably not 'freely' chosen. But if common defences for male circumcision are to be accepted, one could equally hold that since FGC is 'mandated' by strong religious or cultural pressures in some groups, it is something that Western societies ought to tolerate, whereas since FGCS is not 'mandated' in a similar way, it should not be granted this shortcut to tolerance. Either way, the status quo is incoherent.

Simply put, the reasoning deployed to defend preconsensual male circumcision and against preconsensual FGC is sharply at odds with the reasoning deployed to defend adult FGCS and against adult

---

BOX 7.2 Double Standards: A Case Study

This apparent double standard is playing out as we write this chapter. Four members of the Dawoodi Bohra, a small Muslim sect with members in Detroit, Michigan, and other US cities, have recently been indicted on charges of 'Female Genital Mutilation' – the first such case under federal law in the United States [84]. As even opponents of the practice from within the community acknowledge [40], the form of cutting typically practised by the Bohra on their daughters, namely, pricking or excision of a portion of the hood (foreskin) of the external clitoris – often by a doctor in a clinical setting, as in the Detroit case being prosecuted – is significantly less physically invasive than the form of cutting practised by the very same community on their sons, namely, complete removal of the penile foreskin (circumcision). The two forms of cutting may be done at similar ages, for similar reasons; both are regarded as a religious obligation by the Bohra based on similar readings of the same passages of Muslim scripture (in this case, the Hadith – the sayings of the Prophet Mohammed); and both are referred to with the same word, *khatna*. Yet, though the male procedure is more severe, only the female procedure has triggered criminal proceedings under federal law [69].

FGC. In the case of motivations for ritual male circumcision, it is commonly argued that the strength of the associated background norm, whether religious or 'merely' cultural, is a reason for respecting or tolerating the practice, despite the fact that young male children and especially newborn boys are manifestly incapable of providing their own consent. Yet in the case of FGC, the strength of what is in some communities an equally robust and often highly similar background norm is seen as consent-undermining, not only for female minors but also mature adult women – irrespective of their agency or autonomy as might be demonstrated in other contexts.

On one side, then, we have MGC, one form of which is of great religious significance to some groups, while for others it is 'merely' cultural but is not necessarily any less valued. Although it is typically performed on the most intimate part of a child's body before consent can possibly be given or withheld, it is widely accepted and is permitted by Western law. On the other side, we have FGCS, a set of procedures that have primarily aesthetic value for a small – if growing – number of individuals and are of no religious significance to anyone. They are typically performed on adults who are presumed to be competent to provide their own consent but are also increasingly performed on younger girls with the permission (or at the insistence) of their parents. They, too, are relatively uncontroversial and are permitted by Western law. Then in the middle we have FGC, an anatomically overlapping set of procedures performed at various ages, sometimes on adults or older adolescents who are typically presumed, in this case, to be *non*-competent to provide consent, but most often on younger girls with the permission (or at the insistence) of their parents. Certain forms are of great religious significance to some groups *and* have aesthetic value for those who embrace them [86, 87], but all forms are seen as entirely unacceptable, and no form is permitted by Western law.

Explaining the Inconsistencies

Perhaps the difference in attitudes and legislation toward male versus female forms of ritual genital cutting – and between FGC and FGCS – stem not from the religious or cultural significance of one or the other, but from other differences. One common candidate for such a distinction is that FGC – but not FGCS – is performed for reasons that are purely or primarily misogynistic, aiming to curb the sexual lives of girls and women, while male circumcision has no such limiting intention towards boys. As noted recently in the *African Journal of Reproductive Health* [88]:

> Female circumcision has been presented somewhat stereotypically as a practice in which men control female sexuality and female reproduction. The manner in which women have been depicted as victims of a brutal male practice has created sharp reactions, not the least from circumcised women. They have not commonly perceived themselves as victims of a violent male practice but have seen female circumcision as a female custom that is necessary to maintain order [and] to make or create true women.

Consistent with this view, in nearly every culture where FGC occurs it is organised and carried out exclusively by women, with men being barred from participation and often far more likely to report a desire for abandonment of the practice than their female counterparts. Moreover, there is no known community that practices FGC without also practicing MGC, often in parallel and for similar reasons: girls are nowhere being singled out for cutting [9, 56, 89]. By contrast, there are many groups that practise MGC without practising FGC, such as within Judaism, some but not other sects of Islam, and generally in the United States: in those cases, boys *are* singled out for cutting, while girls are strictly protected. Nevertheless, where the two practices do co-occur, prevailing motivations are often close conjugates: ostensible health benefits, aesthetics, religious adherence, hygiene, symbolic entry into adulthood, enhancing one's expected sex appeal, reduction of promiscuity and feminisation or masculinisation of the genitals [90].

Depending on the community in question, any number (or combination) of these and other motivations may apply simultaneously across the gender divide [77]. And while sexual control is sometimes a motivating factor, as we shall discuss, this rationale is not confined to the female rites. In the context of hazing ceremonies, for example, it has been proposed that MGC may be a means by which older males exert sexual dominance over adolescent boys, saying in essence: "We can hurt your penis now, so just think what we can do if you misuse it against us – a warning, if only in symbolic form, of possible castration" [91].

Moreover, in some groups, MGC is explicitly intended to reduce a male's capacity for sexual pleasure. Among the Nso people in Cameroon, for example, one recognised purpose of circumcision is to "tame and moderate the sexual instinct" of men [92]. In addition, the widespread popularity of circumcision in the United States traces directly to historical attempts to curtail masturbation in male children as a form of sexual discipline and 'moral hygiene' [93, 94]. Even today, Western-funded campaigns to circumcise millions of African boys and men as a 'surgical solution' to the spread of HIV are premised in part on the belief that such men cannot be trusted to control their own sexual behaviour (hence the 'need' for surgery):

> Lurking just below the surface in many HIV discussions – especially of HIV in sub-Saharan Africa – is the perception that people in certain countries or regions are more promiscuous, more callous, less empathic, or less moral. Some imply that people living with HIV should abstain from or minimise sexual activity, including reproductive desires.

Thus, some authors have warned that the aggressive Western marketing of male circumcision in such contexts risks reinforcing colonial-era stereotypes about the "sexually promiscuous African male" [95].

None of this detracts from the fact that FGC has, in many cases, become tightly bound up in the regulation of female sexuality, among so many other methods by which such regulation is pursued globally (including FGCS, as we shall argue in a moment). Thus, in some communities, for example in parts of the Sudan, the prizing of female chastity and the subjection of girls and women to the presumed sexual and aesthetic preferences of men are among the primary motivations for FGC [96, 97]. In other communities, "the belief that girls with intact genitalia will be stubborn, promiscuous, or unable to control their sexual desires," or that "genital cutting is necessary [to] prove virginity" may be widespread [20]. In still others, the motives are not primarily anti-sexual, for either females or males [37].

Such variation is only to be expected. As noted by the non-partisan Public Policy Advisory Network on Female Genital Surgeries in Africa, "the vast majority of the world's societies can be described as patriarchal, and most either do not modify the genitals of either sex or modify the genitals of males only. There are almost no patriarchal societies with customary genital surgeries for females only" [9]. Finally, motivations may even differ from family to family. The temptation to universalise over a given motivation should therefore be resisted: the variety of reasons for – and types of – both FGC and MGC across their disparate geographical regions of prevalence frustrate such reductive explanations [9, 37].

Nor should FGCS be permitted to evade critique on this front. Such cosmetic procedures are, by all accounts, largely motivated by a desire for genitals that are perceived to be (a) aesthetically appealing according to restrictive norms propagated within pornography and aided by trends towards total pubic hair removal (which render the genitals more visible), and (b) 'enhanced' in terms of sexual function, which often amounts to the creation of a "tight receptacle for penile penetration" [4]. If there are motivations for FGCS that do not derive from these two main sources, they have not been as well reported. To the extent that both the global pornography industry, and the instrumentalisation of female genitals for penile penetration, are reflections or instantiations of misogyny, it may well be that the motives for FGCS are more universalisable than those for FGC, with as much or more to answer for on this point.

If not health reasons, religious motivations, or misogyny, what is it that makes FGC sufficiently distinct from its close cousins, FGCS and childhood male circumcision, so as to warrant such extreme legislative differences? One possible answer lies beyond medicine or ethics, and instead focusses on the way in which FGC is positioned politically within Western discourses.

Some scholars argue as follows: While male circumcision is more common than FGC within Islam, and there are more circumcised men globally who are Muslim than Jewish, FGC has found itself associated with Islam in ways that have caused the practice to inherit the fears and anxieties created by Islamophobic trends across the Western world [98]. The strength of this association is likely encouraged by the widespread belief that FGC is always performed for sexist or 'patriarchal' reasons, which has contributed to, and meshed with, the vilification of Islam as an inherently misogynistic religion. This framing allows fear of the 'Other' to adopt the more beneficent mask of concern for the welfare of women and girls.

Moreover, unlike the stereotypically imagined recipients of male circumcision (chiefly, Jewish or US American boys) and FGCS (chiefly, white/Western women), FGC is mentally associated almost exclusively with women-of-colour from the Global South. In accordance with the discourses of historical colonial 'civilising missions' and more recent examples of military imperialism, these women are portrayed as lacking autonomy, and as subjugated to the will of their men-folk, thereby impelling Western intervention [99]. The intervention comes in the form of draconian legislation whose primary function is to reassure the public that the perceived 'civilisational threat' is held at bay, and that the ostensible misogyny of *foreign* cultures will not be tolerated.

Meanwhile, because the force of this legislation derives from political rather than ethical narratives, and therefore concentrates on charges of 'barbarism' rather than violations of bodily autonomy per se, male infants as well as intersex children are left unprotected. Further, because these political considerations replace more nuanced inflections within feminist theory and anthropology, cultural norms around female bodies are not brought into the same narrative, leaving FGCS largely free of critique.

In the shadows of these moral lacunae are the women and girls of FGC-prevalent communities, whose diverse needs and perspectives are often lost in the focus on criminality and realpolitik. Unsurprisingly, attitudes towards FGC are as varied as its typology and geographical distribution [20]. While in many regions, a growing minority of women strongly oppose the practice to which they were subjected as children, the more general pattern is that the majority of women within populations of prevalence who have themselves been cut report their continuing support for the practice [100]. Of course, ethics and morality do not reduce to a tally of votes, and beliefs and values can change. But if campaigns to eliminate FGC are ever to be successful, they must take seriously – not condescend towards – the women who do value their cutting traditions, and who regard their modified vulvae as normal or enhanced as opposed to mutilated or otherwise harmed. Meeting such women on their own terms, rather than automatically discounting their perspective or dismissing them as victims of false consciousness, would be a good place to start.

In line with this, despite the variation in typology and culture between regions of prevalence, successful abandonment campaigns share several core features. Among them: centring affected women, engaging local religious or cultural leaders, accommodating the interdependence of communities and their decision-making, showing appropriate respect for cultures, reinforcing their positive aspects and focusing on local values and aspirations [100, 101]. In other words, initiatives which positively engage communities and allow abandonment to be led from within are most likely to be successful. Blanket criminalisation based on double standards, by contrast, is unlikely to foster an atmosphere of cooperation and mutual understanding. Such a realisation has recently led

to calls for legal reform – on practical grounds – even among steadfast anti-FGC advocates [102].

Conclusion

The prevailing view that there is a categorically valid, morally significant difference between the set of acts described as 'FGM' and those known as FGCS is inconsistent with the available evidence concerning both the range of physical interventions constituting such practices, and the cultural and individual motivations behind them. On closer inspection, it is clear that the categories are functional, rather than 'scientific'; they are defined not by the acts they contain (since the physical realities of these acts have considerable overlap), but by the perceived rationales for which they are sought. FGCS acts are sought for purportedly aesthetic reasons (which are themselves rooted in wider cultural norms that deserve scrutiny); FGC acts are sought to adhere to religious or cultural norms (which similarly should be subjected to critique), within which aesthetics is often also a consideration. Even the 'rationale' demarcation is thus evidently blurry.

The more closely one studies the two sets of practices, especially in light of further overlaps with MGC, the greater the apparent similarities between them. Yet acts understood to constitute 'FGM' are criminal, while those within the FGCS category are not. As discussed, one reason for this discrepancy is that the stereotypical reasons for seeking 'FGM' are perceived to be indefensible, while the reasons for seeking FGCS are regarded as less problematic. Moreover, 'FGM' is believed to be primarily (but is not always actually) performed on children, who cannot give consent, while FGCS is believed to be primarily (but is not always actually) sought by adults, who (contestably) can. But even if such presumed distinctions were more strongly rooted in reality, they would be undermined by the fact that religious or cultural male circumcision – which is more physically invasive than at least some prohibited forms of FGC – is legal almost everywhere, often unregulated, and primarily performed on infants and newborns who are least capable of consenting.

Given such inconsistencies, it is increasingly being argued that the laws concerning genital alteration are not based in objective or universally valid distinctions, but are rather heavily shaped by certain social and political discourses regarding race and gender [83]. This creates a confusing situation for medical professionals, whose work requires a clear understanding of the differences between the two practices, yet the (largely unexplained) division offered by the law is not derivable from, nor consistent with, the tenets of medical ethics [103].

Changes to legislation around genital alteration in Western contexts could be approached in several ways. Some would argue that, in liberal, multicultural societies, it is important to permit pluralism in the law in order to accommodate the practices of minority ethnic and religious groups, even if those practices involve irreversible modifications to the bodies of children. On that view, one might argue that the law around FGC (perhaps with certain typological restrictions) should be brought into line with its parallel practice, MGC [65]. Others would contend that the only defensible distinction is that between those who have the capacity to consent, and those who do not, and that if pluralism in the law should be upheld, it should be reserved for the bodies of adults [82]. Such a view motivates changes to the law according to which non-therapeutic genital alterations are unlawful for all children, and lawful for all adults [33, 61]. This would allow genital surgeries to be chosen, if desired, on the basis of one's own mature preferences and values, regardless of race or gender, and to be offered within regulated clinical conditions with due attention to possible complications and follow-up care.

References

1. Weston J. Female genital mutilation: The law as it relates to children. *Arch Dis Child.* 2017;102(9):864–7.

2. Liao LM, Creighton SM. Requests for cosmetic genitoplasty: How should healthcare providers respond? *BMJ* 2007;334(7603):1090.

3. Liao LM, Taghinejadi N, Creighton SM. An analysis of the content and clinical implications of online advertisements for female genital cosmetic surgery. *BMJ Open.* 2012;2(6):e001908.

4. Rodrigues S. From vaginal exception to exceptional vagina: The biopolitics of female genital cosmetic surgery. *Sexualities.* 2012;15(7):778–94.

5. Kadian YS, Pradeep K, Verma V. Feminizing genitoplasty in congenital adrenal hyperplasia: A new method for clitoral reduction. *Arch Int Surg.* 2016;6(3):153–7.

6. Ehrenreich N, Barr M. Intersex surgery, female genital cutting, and the selective condemnation of "cultural practices." *Harv CR-CL Law Rev.* 2005;40(1):71–140.

7. Davis DS. Male and female genital alteration: A collision course with the law. *Health Matrix.* 2001;11:487–570.

8. Abusharaf RM. Virtuous cuts: Female genital circumcision in an African ontology. *Differences.* 2001;12(1):112–40.

9. Abdulcadir J, Ahmadu FS, Catania L, et al. Seven things to know about female genital surgeries in Africa. *Hastings Center Rep.* 2012;42(6):19–27.

10. WHO/UN. Eliminating female genital mutilation: An interagency statement. Geneva: World Health Organization. 2008. Available from: www.un.org/womenwatch/daw/csw/csw52/statements_missions/Interagency_Statement_on_Eliminating_FGM.pdf

11. Stewart PJ, Strathern A., eds. *Ritual.* London: Routledge; 2017.

12. Taylor JR, Lockwood AP, Taylor AJ. The prepuce: Specialized mucosa of the penis and its loss to circumcision. *BJU Int.* 1996;77(2):291–5.

13. Wilcken A, Keil T, Dick B. Traditional male circumcision in eastern and southern Africa: A systematic review of prevalence and complications. *Bull WHO.* 2010;88(12):907–14.

14. Ramos S, Boyle GJ. Ritual and medical circumcision among Filipino boys. In Denniston GC, Hodges FM, Milos MF (eds), *Understanding circumcision.* New York: Springer; 2001, pp. 253–70.

15. Glass M. Forced circumcision of men (abridged). *J Med Ethics.* 2014;40(8):567–71.

16. Pounder DJ. Ritual mutilation: Subincision of the penis among Australian Aborigines. *Am J Forensic Med Pathol.* 1983;4(3):227–30.

17. Rickwood AM. Medical indications for circumcision. *BJU Int.* 1999;83(S1):45–51.

18. Wallerstein E. Circumcision: The uniquely American medical enigma. *Urol Clin North Am.* 1985;12(1):123–32.

19. Hofvander Y. New law on male circumcision in Sweden. *Lancet.* 2002;359(9306):630.

20. Earp BD, Sardi LM, Jellison WA. False beliefs predict increased circumcision satisfaction in a sample of US American men. *Cult Health Sex.* 2018;20(8):945-955.

21. Hammond T, Carmack A. Long-term adverse outcomes from neonatal circumcision reported in a survey of 1,008 men: An overview of health and human rights implications. *Int J Hum Rights.* 2017;21(2):189–218.

22. Ball PJ. A survey of subjective foreskin sensation in 600 intact men. In Denniston GC, Grassivaro Gallo P, Hodges FM, Milos MF, Viviani F (eds), *Bodily integrity and the politics of circumcision.* Dordrecht: Springer; 2006, pp. 177–88.

23. Bossio JA, Pukall CF, Steele SS. Examining penile sensitivity in neonatally circumcised and intact men using quantitative sensory testing. *J Urol.* 2016;195(6): 1848–53.

24. Frisch M, Simonsen J. Cultural background, non-therapeutic circumcision and the risk of meatal stenosis and other urethral stricture disease: Two nationwide register-based cohort studies in Denmark 1977–2013. *Surgeon.* 2018;16(2):107–118.

25. Krill AJ, Palmer LS, Palmer JS. Complications of circumcision. *Sci World J.* 2011;11:2458–68.

26. Earp BD, Allareddy V, Rotta AT. Factors associated with early deaths following neonatal male circumcision in the United States, 2001–2010. *Clinical Pediatrics.* 2018;57 (13):1532–1540.

27. Gonzalez L. South Africa: Over half a million initiates maimed under the knife. All Africa. 2014; June 25. Available from: www.health-e.org.za/2014/06/25/half-million-initiates-maimed-knife/

28. Mabuza W. Report on public hearings on male initiation schools in South Africa, 2010. Commission for the Protection and Promotion of the Rights of Cultural, Religious and Linguistic Communities. Report 978-0-620-51683-9 (pp. 1–77). 2010. Available from: www.health-e.org.za/wp-content/uploads/2014/06/CRL-Report-on-Public-Hearings-on-Male-Initiation-Schools-in-South-Africa.pdf

29. Tobian AA, Gray RH. The medical benefits of male circumcision. *JAMA.* 2011;306(13):1479–80.

30. Bossio JA, Pukall CF, Steele S. A review of the current state of the male circumcision literature. *J Sex Med.* 2014;11(12):2847–64.

31. Frisch M, Earp BD. Circumcision of male infants and children as a public health measure in developed countries: A critical assessment of recent evidence. *Global Public Health.* 2016. 2018;13(5):626–641.

32. Saito S, Hata H, Inamura Y, Kitamura S, Yanagi T, Shimizu H. Vulvar basal cell carcinoma with adhesion of the labia majora and minora. *Clin Exp Dermatol.* 2017;42(1):92–3.

33. Mason C. Exorcising excision: Medico-legal issues arising from male and female genital surgery in Australia. *J Law Med.* 2001;9(1):58–67.

34. Shell-Duncan B, Hernlund Y, eds. *Female "circumcision" in Africa: Culture, controversy, and change.* Boulder, CO: Lynne Rienner; 2000.

35. Shahvisi A. Cutting slack and cutting corners: An ethical and pragmatic response to Arora and Jacobs' "Female genital alteration: A compromise solution." *J Med Ethics.* 2016;42(3):156–7.

36. Fahmy A, El-Mouelhy MT, Ragab AR. Female genital mutilation/cutting and issues of sexuality in Egypt. *Reprod Health Matters.* 2010;18(36): 181–90.

37. Leonard L. Interpreting female genital cutting: Moving beyond the impasse. *Ann Rev Sex Res.* 2000;11(1): 158–90.

38. Merli C. Sunat for girls in southern Thailand: Its relation to traditional midwifery, male circumcision and other obstetrical practices. *Finn J Ethnic Migrat.* 2008;3(2):32–41.

39. Merli C. Male and female genital cutting among Southern Thailand's Muslims: Rituals, biomedical practice and local discourses. *Cult Health Sex.* 2010;12 (7):725–38.

40. Taher M. Understanding FGM in the Dawoodi Bohra community: An exploratory study. Sahiyo. 2017. Available from: https://sahiyo.files.wordpress.com/2017/02/sahiyo_report_final-updatedbymt2.pdf

41. WHO. Classification of female genital mutilation. World Health Organization. 2017. Available from: www.who.int/reproductivehealth/topics/fgm/overview/en/

42. Hamori CA. Aesthetic surgery of the female genitalia: Labiaplasty and beyond. *Plast Reconstruct Surg.* 2014;134(4):661–73.

43. Rodriguez, SB. *Female circumcision and clitoridectomy in the United States: a history of a medical treatment.* Rochester, NY: University of Rochester Press; 2014.

44. Veale D, Daniels J. Cosmetic clitoridectomy in a 33-year-old woman. *Arch Sex Behav.* 2012;41(3):725–30.

45. Committee on Gynecologic Practice, American College of Obstetricians and Gynecologists. ACOG Committee Opinion No 378: "Vaginal rejuvenation" and cosmetic vaginal procedures. *Obstet Gynecol.* 2007;110(3):737.

46. Earp BD. Hymen "restoration" in cultures of oppression: How can physicians promote individual patient welfare without becoming complicit in the perpetuation of unjust social norms? *J Med Ethics.* 2013;40(6):431.

47. Millner VS, Eichold BH, Sharpe TH, Lynn SC. First glimpse of the functional benefits of clitoral hood piercings. *Am J Obstet Gynecol.* 2005;193(3):675–6.

48. Narain S, Eva L, Luesley D. A rare case of pseudolymphoma of the vulva. *J Obstet Gynaecol.* 2009;29(3):254–5.

49. Mowat H, McDonald K, Dobson AS, Fisher J, Kirkman M. The contribution of online content to the promotion and normalisation of female genital

cosmetic surgery: A systematic review of the literature. *BMC Womens Health*. 2015;15(110):1–10.

50. UNICEF. Female genital mutilation/cutting: A statistical overview and exploration of the dynamics of change. UNICEF. 2013. Available from: www .unicef.org/media/files/UNICEF_FGM_report_July _2013_Hi_res.pdf

51. Conroy, RM. Female genital mutilation: Whose problem, whose solution? *BMJ*. 2006;333(7559):106–7.

52. Kaefer M, Rink RC. Treatment of the enlarged clitoris. *Front Pediatr*. 2017;5(125):1–11.

53. Catania L, Abdulcadir O, Puppo V, Verde JB, Abdulcadir J, Abdulcadir D. Pleasure and orgasm in women with female genital mutilation/cutting (FGM/C). *J Sex Med*. 2007;4(6):1666–78.

54. Pearce AJ, Bewley S. Medicalization of female genital mutilation: Harm reduction or unethical? *Obstet Gynaecol Reprod Med*. 2014;24(1):29–30.

55. Arie S. Cosmetic industry regulation is only skin deep. *BMJ Online*. 2017;357(j3047):1–2.

56. Earp BD. Between moral relativism and moral hypocrisy: Reframing the debate on "FGM." *Kennedy Inst Ethics J*. 2016;26(2):105–44.

57. Wood PL. Cosmetic genital surgery in children and adolescents. *Best Practice & Res Clin Obstet Gynaecol*. 2018;48(1):137–146.

58. Kelly B, Foster C. Should female genital cosmetic surgery and genital piercing be regarded ethically and legally as female genital mutilation? *BJOG*. 2012;119 (4):389–92.

59. Johnsdotter S, Mestre RM. Female genital mutilation in Europe: An analysis of court cases. 2015. Available from: https://publications.europa.eu/en/publication-d etail/-/publication/7fff7a7b-fc84-11e5-b713-01aa75e d71a1/language-en

60. Female Genital Mutilation Act 2003. Available from: www.legislation.gov.uk/ukpga/2003/31/pdfs/ukp ga_20030031_en.pdf

61. Dustin M. Female genital mutilation/cutting in the UK: Challenging the inconsistencies. *Eur J Womens Stud*. 2010;17(1):7–23.

62. Crouch NS, Deans R, Michala L, Liao LM, Creighton SM. Clinical characteristics of well women seeking labial reduction surgery: A prospective study. *BJOG*. 2011;118(12):1507–10.

63. Edwards A. What is the dynamic between the "cosmetic versus cultural surgery" discourse and efforts to end FGM in the UK? 2013. Dissertation, Oxford Brookes University. Available from: www .halsburyslawexchange.co.uk/wp-content/uploads/site s/25/2015/03/Alice_Edwards_Dissertation_Dec_13_F GM.pdf

64. Shahvisi, A. Female genital mutilation and cultural pluralism: Racism, sexism and hypocrisy. In Kuehlmeyer K, Odukoya D, Klingler C, Huxtable R (eds), *Ethical, legal and social aspects of healthcare for migrants: Perspectives from the UK and Germany*. London: Routledge; 2018.

65. Arora KS, Jacobs AJ. Female genital alteration: A compromise solution. *J Med Ethics*. 2016;42(3): 148–54.

66. Goodman MP, Placik OJ, Benson III RH, et al. A large multicenter outcome study of female genital plastic surgery. *J Sex Med*. 2010;7(4):1565–77.

67. British Medical Association. Female genital mutilation: Caring for patients and safeguarding children. 2011. BMA: London. Available from: www .bma.org.uk/-media/files/pdfs/practical%20advice%20 at%20work/ethics/femalegenitalmutilation.pdf

68. Leye E, Ysebaert I, Deblonde J, et al. Female genital mutilation: Knowledge, attitudes and practices of Flemish gynaecologists. *Eur J Contracept Reprod Health Care*. 2008;13(2):182–90.

69. Earp, BD. Does female genital mutilation have health benefits? The problem with medicalizing morality. Quillette. 2017. Available from: http://quillette.com/ 2017/08/15/female-genital-mutilation-health-benefits- problem-medicalizing-morality/

70. Shweder RA. The goose and the gander: The genital wars. *Global Discourse*. 2013;3(2):348–66.

71. Earp BD. Infant circumcision and adult penile sensitivity: Implications for sexual experience. *Trends Urol Mens Health*. 2016;7(4):17–21.

72. Mackenzie C. On bodily autonomy. In Toombs SK (ed), *Handbook of phenomenology and medicine*. Dordrecht: Springer; 2001, pp. 417–439.

73. Mazor J. The child's interests and the case for the permissibility of male infant circumcision. *J Med Ethics*. 2013;39(7):421–8.

74. Darby RJ. The child's right to an open future: Is the principle applicable to non-therapeutic circumcision? *J Med Ethics*. 2013;39(7):463–8.

75. Earp BD, Darby R. Circumcision, sexual experience, and harm. *U Penn J Int Law*. 2017;37(2–online), 1–56.

76. Myers A. Neonatal male circumcision, if not already commonplace, would be plainly unacceptable by modern ethical standards. *Am J Bioethics*. 2015;15(2): 54–5.

77. Brusa M, Barilan YM. Cultural circumcision in EU public hospitals: An ethical discussion. *Bioethics*. 2009;23(8):470–82.

78. WHO. Male circumcision: Global trends and determinants of prevalence, safety and acceptability. World Health Organization. 2007. Available from:

http://apps.who.int/iris/bitstream/10665/43749/1/978
9241596169_eng.pdf

79. Goodman J. Jewish circumcision: An alternative perspective. *BJU Int.* 1999;83(S1):2–7.

80. Xu B, Goldman H. Newborn circumcision in Victoria, Australia: Reasons and parental attitudes. *ANZ J Surg.* 2008;78(11):1019–22.

81. Jacobs AJ, Arora KS. Punishment of minor female genital ritual procedures: Is the perfect the enemy of the good? *Dev World Bioethics.* 2017;17(2): 134–40.

82. Earp BD. In defence of genital autonomy for children. *J Med Ethics.* 2016;42(3):158–63.

83. Earp BD, Hendry J, Thomson M. Reason and paradox in medical and family law: Shaping children's bodies. *Med Law Rev.* 2017;25(4):604–27.

84. Belluck P. Michigan case adds U.S. dimension to debate on genital mutilation. *New York Times.* 2017. Available from: www.nytimes.com/2017/06/10/health/genital-mutilation-muslim-dawoodi-bohra-michigan-case.html

85. Veale D. Reply to Bewley (2012). *Arch Sex Behav.* 2013;42(3):325.

86. Manderson L. Local rites and body politics: Tensions between cultural diversity and human rights. *Int Feminist J Politics.* 2004;6(2):285–307.

87. Ahmadu FS, Shweder RA. Disputing the myth of the sexual dysfunction of circumcised women: An interview with Fuambai S. Ahmadu by Richard A. Shweder. *Anthropol Today.* 2009;25(6):14–7.

88. Vestbostad E, Blystad A. Reflections on female circumcision discourse in Hargeysa, Somaliland: Purified or mutilated? *Afr J Reprod Health.* 2014;18 (2):22–35.

89. Shweder RA. What about "female genital mutilation"? And why understanding culture matters in the first place. *Daedalus.* 2000;129(4):209–32.

90. Svoboda JS. Promoting genital autonomy by exploring commonalities between male, female, intersex, and cosmetic female genital cutting. *Global Discourse.* 2013;3(2):237–55.

91. Schlegel A, Barry H III. Pain, fear, and circumcision in boys' adolescent initiation ceremonies. *Cross Cult Res.* 2017; 1069397116685780.

92. Hellsten SK. Rationalising circumcision: From tradition to fashion, from public health to individual freedom – critical notes on cultural persistence of the practice of genital mutilation. *J Med Ethics.* 2004;30(3):248–53.

93. Aggleton P. "Just a snip"? A social history of male circumcision. *Reprod Health Matters.* 2007;15 (29):15–21.

94. Darby R. *A surgical temptation: The demonization of the foreskin and the rise of circumcision in Britain.* Chicago: University of Chicago Press; 2013.

95. Sawires SR, Dworkin SL, Fiamma A, Peacock D, Szekeres G, Coates TJ. Male circumcision and HIV/AIDS: Challenges and opportunities. *Lancet.* 2007;369(9562):708–13.

96. Almroth L, Almroth-Berggren V, Hassanein OM, et al. A community based study on the change of practice of female genital mutilation in a Sudanese village. *Int J Gynecol Obstet.* 2001;74(2):179–85.

97. Lowenstein LF. Attitudes and attitude differences to female genital mutilation in the Sudan: Is there a change on the horizon? *Soc Sci Med A: Med Psychol Med Sociol.* 1978;12:417–21.

98. Morgan G. *Global Islamophobia: Muslims and moral panic in the West.* London: Routledge; 2016.

99. Spivak GC. Can the subaltern speak? In Morris R (ed), *Can the subaltern speak? Reflections on the history of an idea.* New York: Columbia University Press; 1998/ 2010, pp. 21–78.

100. UNICEF. The dynamics of social change towards the abandonment of female genital mutilation/cutting in five African countries. UNICEF. 2010. Available from; www.unicef-irc.org/publications/pdf/fgm_insight_eng.pdf

101. Johansen RE, Diop NJ, Laverack G, Leye E. What works and what does not: A discussion of popular approaches for the abandonment of female genital mutilation. *Obstet Gynecol Int.* 2013;2013(348248):1–10.

102. Townley L, Bewley S. Why the law against female genital mutilation should be scrapped. The Conversation. 2017. Available from: https://theconversation.com/why-the-law-against-female-genital-mutilation-should-be-scrapped-79851

103. Shahvisi A. Why UK doctors should be troubled by female genital mutilation legislation. *Clin Ethics.* 2016;12(2):102–8.

Choice and Female Genital Cosmetic Surgery

Clare Chambers

I google 'labiaplasty'.[1] The first result is for "MYA Labiaplasty – Join 1000s of Happy Patients." Clicking on the link, I learn:

> Labiaplasty is MYA's most popular vaginal surgery and makes up 97% of procedures. For women after a quick procedure with effective results that will boost confidence and comfort, labia surgery is an excellent choice which forms part of our popular designer vagina surgery options. [2]

Back to Google. The next result is "Labiaplasty Surgery – 40 min Out Patient Procedure". This link takes me to The Surrey Park Clinic, which opens with:

> Many women feel discomfort or embarrassment if the labia minora (the inner lips of the vulva) are enlarged. This can affect quality of life by causing worry about what clothes to wear and intimate relationships. Sometimes the fear of negative comments can affect the confidence of women and can even put them off starting a relationship. Surgical correction is a very straightforward procedure and the impact it can have on a woman's self esteem can be profound. [3]

The third entry is for the Medico Beauty Clinic. Their information about labiaplasty also signals the normality of the procedure:

> Many women dislike the large protuberant appearance of their labia minora and wish to change their appearance. In some instances, women with large labia can experience pain during intercourse, or feel

discomfort during everyday activities or when wearing tight-fitting clothing. Others may feel unattractive, or wish to enhance their sexual experiences by removing some of the skin that covers the clitoris. [4]

In each case, the providers of female genital cosmetic surgery (FGCS) signal the advantages of the procedure and give a number of reasons why it might be a desirable *choice*. Most prominently cite the negative feelings that FGCS can remove: fear, worry, embarrassment, pain, discomfort, dislike and feeling unattractive. Less prominent are the positives: boosting confidence and comfort, creating a 'designer vagina', increasing self-esteem and enhancing sexual experiences. But the overall message, as MYA clinic concludes, is that "labia surgery is an excellent choice."

In this chapter I challenge the idea that an appeal to choice exonerates FGCS. My argument proceeds in five stages. First, I consider the normative role that choice plays in liberal society and philosophy. Second, I note that UK law does not treat choice as adequate for accessing FGCS. Third, I consider the relationship between choice and the concept of normality. Fourth, I consider choice in the context of cosmetic surgery generally, and analyse the distinctive features of FGCS. Fifth, I consider the policy implications of my analysis.

Choice as a Normative Transformer

In liberal democracies there is a general presumption that individuals should be left free to choose whether to participate in practices that affect only themselves. One key proponent of this idea is philosopher John Stuart Mill, who writes: "The only part of the conduct of any one, for which he is amenable to society, is that which concerns others. In the part which merely concerns himself, his independence is, of right, absolute. Over himself, over his own body and mind, the individual is sovereign" [5, p. 78]. This presumption of individual freedom of choice suggests the permissibility of cosmetic surgery. If people want to undergo surgical procedures

---

[1] Labiaplasty is not the only form of female genital cosmetic surgery (FGCS) but it is the most common and well known. The Royal College of Obstetricians and Gynaecologists (RCOG) defines FGCS as follows: "FGCS refers to non-medically indicated cosmetic surgical procedures which change the structure and appearance of the healthy external genitalia of women, or internally in the case of vaginal tightening. This definition includes the most common procedure, labiaplasty, as well as others, such as hymenoplasty and vaginoplasty, also known as vaginal reconstruction and vaginal rejuvenation." See [1], p. 1.

to alter their body they should be free to do so, and it would be beyond the scope of the liberal state to forbid them. Prioritising choice thus supports the legalisation of all forms of surgical modification on everyone capable of exercising choice.

Mill is by no means the only philosopher to prioritise choice. Many political philosophers use choice as what I call a 'normative transformer'. A normative transformer is something that changes an outcome from normatively unacceptable to normatively acceptable [6]. Choice may be used to normatively transform an inequality from one that is unjust to one that is just. For example, some theorists argue that it is not an injustice if women are paid less than men so long as the reason for this pay gap is that women and men choose different jobs [7]. Or choice may be used to normatively transform a criminal assault into a legal act, as when rape is criminalised but even violent consensual sex is not, or when boxing is legal but grievous bodily harm (GBH) is not, or when consensual surgery is legal but non-consensual surgery is not. Choice may also be used as a normative transformer in a more general sense, indicating that a practice should be immune from moral or other judgement if it has been chosen. One example is the idea that feminism means not criticising women's choices, even if they choose to participate in gendered practices such as cosmetic surgery, wearing makeup, or removing body hair [8].

Although Mill's principle of individual choice is extremely influential and generally accepted, it is usually thought to admit of exceptions. Most states do engage in some forms of paternalism, forbidding their citizens from making some choices for their own good. For example, it is common for even liberal states to require the use of seatbelts in cars or to forbid the use of dangerous recreational drugs. Paternalism in cases such as these may be justified by the seriousness of the harm that paternalism prevents, or by factors that undermine the extent to which individuals can really be said to be choosing freely.

Elsewhere I have argued that there are grounds for state interference in individuals' choices if those choices are characterised by both *disadvantage* and *influence*. [6] The disadvantage factor applies if a choice disadvantages those who make it, relative to those who choose differently. This disadvantage may be physical or mental, such as the risk of bodily harm or emotional distress. Alternatively, the disadvantage may be economic or status-based, such as suffering

financial cost or being regarded as inferior. The disadvantage factor alerts us to the fact that if people make choices that disadvantage them, there is a prima facie reason to be concerned about that choice.

The second factor that prevents choice from properly acting as a normative transformer is the influence factor. The influence factor applies if there are identifiable pressures on the choosers to choose as they do. This influence may be direct and interpersonal, such as when a man repeatedly tells his partner that she would look better with breast implants. Or it may be more diffuse and capillary, such as when women live in a general climate of focus on their appearance, with magazines, adverts and beauty products combining to portray an image of the ideal or even acceptable woman [6, 9, 10]. If the influence factor is present then we should question whether the choice really is a free one.

The influence factor on its own is not enough to render a choice suspect. All choices are made within a social context. All of us form our preferences and shape our choices around the norms and expectations of that context. But where there are identifiable ways in which people are pressured to make choices that disadvantage them – that is, where the influence and disadvantage factors are combined – there is reason to think that choice should not be regarded as a normative transformer. Choices that are characterised by disadvantage and influence are cases of injustice, and may justify intervention from the state and other actors.

FGCS and the Law

UK law does not grant women permission to undergo genital procedures whenever they choose. The practice of genital cutting, known legally as female genital mutilation (FGM), is outlawed, even for consenting adult women, by the UK Female Genital Mutilation Act 2003. The Act states, "It is a criminal offence to excise, infibulate or otherwise mutilate the whole or any part of a girl's labia majora, labia minora or clitoris."

The primary justification for this prohibition is that FGM is a harmful, dangerous and destructive practice that paradigmatically involves the mutilation of young girls against their will in order to satisfy sexist cultural norms. Women and girls therefore need to be protected from the practice by legal prohibition. This case for outlawing FGM performed on girls under the age of 18 can follow a simple choice-based logic, without invoking the analysis I offered earlier. Children are commonly not thought to have the ability to give consent on serious, irreversible, risky procedures such as FGM, for two reasons. First, children lack the mental capacity to gather adequate information and assess it rationally. Second, children lack the ability to withhold consent because they are under the effective control of parents and other adults, meaning that they are likely to cave in to pressure to consent to procedures they do not want, or that they are vulnerable to sanction and abuse if they do manage to resist. So, an approach that prioritises choice is consistent with the illegality of FGM for children. Indeed, an approach of this kind has implications that extend far beyond the existing legal framework, as it implies the impermissibility of many cultural and cosmetic practices routinely performed on children such as male circumcision, otoplasty and cosmetic dentistry.[2]

However, while the UK Female Genital Mutilation Act 2003 refers to "girls", its provisions also apply to adult women. That is to say, the Act explicitly prevents any woman from choosing modification of her genitals without clinical indication. This prohibition includes labiaplasty and other similar procedures, as labiaplasty just is to "excise … part of a girl's labia majora [or] labia minora." Labiaplasty is thus explicitly covered by the definition of procedures that are presumptively illegal under the Female Genital Mutilation Act.[3]

However, FGCS is widely available in the UK, and openly advertised, as we saw at the start of this chapter. This is possible because the Act allows an exception: "no offence is committed by an approved person who performs a surgical operation on a girl which is necessary for her physical or mental health." There are restrictions on what sorts of things count as making surgery *necessary*: the Act stipulates, "For the purpose

of determining whether an operation is necessary for the mental health of a girl it is immaterial whether she or any other person believes that the operation is required as a matter of custom or ritual" [14]. However, the guidance notes for the legislation say that procedures that are necessary for mental health can include "cosmetic surgery resulting from the distress caused by a perception of abnormality." [15]

This perception of abnormality does not have to be based on fact; it is legal to operate on genitals that are perfectly normal. For labiaplasty to be legal, all that is needed is that women choosing it should *think* that their labia are abnormal, so that this perception causes them sufficient distress as to constitute (or be portrayed as) a barrier to mental health. The result is that FGM is ruled out absolutely, even if genuinely freely chosen by an adult woman, but labiaplasty is permissible if it can be shown to be *necessary* for the patient's mental health. In practice, FGCS is performed without legal sanction not only on adult women but also on children, meaning that parents are able to authorise FGM on their daughters if it is justified by aesthetics but not if it is justified by tradition.

Now, none of the foregoing adverts for FGCS explicitly refer to mental health, or state that they are able to operate only on patients with a mental health problem. The "distress caused by the perception of abnormality" wording allows women to access FGCS merely on the basis of choice, in practice. But that is not its intention. FGCS is legal in the UK only if the distress is sufficient to constitute diminished mental health. In other words, for FGCS to be legal, women have to be suffering. But surgery does not have to be the only way to alleviate their suffering. The Act merely requires that women's distress be caused by the *perception* of abnormality; actual abnormality or pathology is not required. This wording may explain the predominance of negativity in the FGCS providers' marketing material. The joyous 'designer vaginas' of MYA are on shakier ground.

Choosing to Be Normal

The desire to be normal is a crucial part of many patients' decisions to undergo cosmetic surgery, whatever the procedure [6, 9, 16]. Commercial cosmetic surgery providers therefore benefit from encouraging prospective patients to think that their natural bodies are abnormal. They are ably assisted in this marketing strategy by a vast industry of beauty, fashion, media

---

[2] For a charity that campaigns against unnecessary genital cutting of children, whether male, female, or intersex, see Future Choices at www.futurechoices.org.uk. For a report criticising cosmetic procedures on children and calling for them to be banned outside the context of multidisciplinary health care see [9].

[3] Speaking as Home Secretary, Teresa May stated in 2014 that FGCS is outlawed by the 2003 Act [11]. Legal firm Mills & Reeve refers to female genital cosmetic surgery as "technically unlawful" [12, p. 1]. Marge Berer notes that, in the UK, "there is a law against female genital mutilation (FGM) which describes it in the very same terms as the procedure described by the Department of Health as labia reduction" [13].

including social media, and pornography, all problematising the normal body – particularly if that body is female [1, 17]. For FGCS providers the stakes are particularly high: the legality of the practice depends on women thinking they are abnormal, and on that perception causing them significant distress. Because a vast range in the size of the labia minora is in fact perfectly normal [18], and the vast majority of women seeking FGCS fall within normal range [1, 19, 20], commercial providers of FGCS rely on women being falsely persuaded that there is something wrong with their genitals.

As we saw at the start of this chapter, FGCS providers often market the procedure by encouraging prospective patients to think that there is something wrong with their genitals. The providers refer to the "many women" who are distressed by their labia and highlight the popularity of FGCS. The paradoxical nature of the idea that it could be normal to have abnormal genitals does not matter if all that is needed is a *perception* of abnormality. The providers of FGCS thus present the *surgery* as normal and the natural female *body* as abnormal.

What counts as normal thus becomes a matter of subjective rather than objective fact, a matter of social norms rather than anatomical reality. Choosing to be normal is thus about choosing to conform to social norms rather than choosing to rectify clinical abnormality. The choice to be normal, like choice more generally, is *socially constructed*.

Social construction can be divided into two phenomena: the social construction of *options* and the social construction of *preferences*. Consider first the social construction of options. For an option to be chosen, that option has to be available as an option in the social context of the chooser. Labiaplasty and other forms of FCGS are relatively new procedures and their popularity has risen rapidly [9, 20]. Women can choose to undergo FGCS only if that procedure exists, technologically, and if surgeons are willing to perform it. The choice to undergo FGCS also requires GPs who are willing to recommend it and refer patients for it, or marketing to make commercial patients aware of it. It may also require the availability of finance for the procedure. All these factors are social: they depend on a particular social context in which FGCS is normalised and the natural vulva is pathologised.

The second aspect of the social construction of choice is the social construction of preferences. Women have to want FGCS if they are to choose it.

For FGCS to be appealing, then the benefits it offers or the problems it alleviates have to seem more important than the costs it entails. The costs of FGCS are fairly straightforward: they include financial cost; the time spent in consultations, surgery and recovery; the pain caused by the procedure; the loss of highly sensitive erogenous tissue; and the risk of complications. The choice to undergo FGCS may involve an active attempt to minimise those costs – or, more precisely, to minimise patients' awareness of the extent of those costs. There is evidence that cosmetic surgery providers do not always adequately ensure that their patients are fully aware of the costs and risks of procedures and that, even where they do, the message does not always get across [9].[4] Certainly the value of intact labia is not emphasised. As an example, note the idea in the Medico Beauty Clinic website extract, quoted earlier, that labiaplasty removes skin that gets in the way of sexual pleasure, rather than that skin itself being a source of sexual pleasure.

But the choice to undergo FGCS also requires a sense that the procedure will be beneficial. For cosmetic surgery in general, and for FGCS in particular, the advantages are fundamentally socially constructed. FGCS has increased in popularity extremely rapidly, coinciding with the increased ubiquity of pornography, viewed online, and an accompanying strong norm that women should remove all their pubic hair [17, 22, 23]. These very recent changes provide the social conditions for the perception of labial abnormality. It is not surprising that women develop the sense that their labia are abnormal only in social conditions in which it is easy to view many other women's labia, in pornography and unobscured by pubic hair [24, 25].

What is normal thus depends not simply on what is numerically common, or on what is non-pathological, or on what is well-functioning. The labia of women who choose labiaplasty are most likely neither uncommonly large, nor pathological, nor dysfunctional. What is normal is culturally relative. It may also depend on ignorance of the true prevalence of a particular trait, an ignorance that may be accidental or cultivated. Women *can* be concerned about the normality of their genitals without viewing pornography or adverts for cosmetic surgery: if a body part is deeply private, even taboo,

---

[4] Lauren Greenfield's photographs of women undergoing and recovering from cosmetic surgery allude to the fact that patients would rather not think about what the surgery actually involves. See [21].

then the lack of exemplars of that part can lead to ignorance, anxiety and doubt. In these contexts, increased visibility leads to a broadening of the concept of normality. But the increased visibility of vulvas in ever-more-accessible pornography (including the vulvas of women who have had FGCS), the norm for complete pubic hair removal and the intensive marketing of FGCS all lead to a narrowing of the concept of normal.[5] Self-esteem, confidence and embarrassment are all emotions that relate intricately to social context.

Even those benefits of FGCS that relate to physical experience are socially dependent. Some women have FGCS to avoid the pain of tight trousers.[6] If tight trousers were not fashionable for women, this problem would probably not arise. Once it does arise, the decision to solve it with FGCS rather than different clothes makes sense only in a social context in which women are encouraged to think of their bodies as naturally deficient, and in which women routinely are expected to place their appearance above their comfort and choose how they *look* over how they *feel* or how they *are*.

The fact that the benefits of FGCS are socially constructed does not mean that they are not real. That is to say, given the social costs and benefits of the practice in any particular context, it may be rational for an individual woman to choose FGCS. For her, it may be a surgery that makes sense to choose. But to make an assessment of the normative features of that choice – to know whether choice is properly treated as a normative transformer in this case – the question is: what social conditions have to be in place to make this choice a rational or comprehensible one?

In the case of FGCS, the social conditions required to make sense of the practice include the social value denied to women, the primacy attributed to women's appearance, the centring of the pornographic, the subordination of women's erogenous experience to their sexual confidence, the commercialisation of low self-esteem and the conscious and cynical manipulation of anxiety. FGCS will be chosen by women if they are encouraged to see deformity rather than beauty, and to seek solace in the scalpel.

The Disadvantage and Influence of FGCS

FGCS is a choice that is characterised by both the influence and the disadvantage factors. It is a choice that women face significant pressure to make. This pressure comes from the images of vulvas they see in pornography and the internet, or from comments by men who have seen cosmetically modified vulvas in pornography, or from the normalisation of the practice when it is discussed in the mainstream media, or from parents who are concerned that their daughters' genitals look different, or from GPs and other health care providers who recommend FCGS as a 'solution' for genitals that are perfectly normal or from the marketing materials offered by FGCS providers.[7]

But it is also a choice that puts women at a disadvantage, compared to men or to women who do not undergo genital surgery. All surgery brings with it pain and the risk of side effects, and requires recovery time. FGCS is no exception, and also involves the removal of highly sensitive irreplaceable erogenous tissue. Like all commercial surgery, FGCS involves financial cost. All these costs of FGCS can be regarded as disadvantages that accrue to those who choose it.

But FGCS involves another disadvantage, which is that it requires the woman who chooses it to think that her natural body is deformed or deficient, and that surgery is required to rectify it. All cosmetic surgery may involve this feature. But FGCS is distinctive in that it requires the perception of one's own abnormality as a condition of legality of the surgery, and so it is a perception that providers are bound to encourage. It is a severe disadvantage of status to be encouraged to believe that one's own body is abnormal.

---

[5] For example, Gemma Sharp, Julie Mattiske and Kirstin I. Vale found that the majority of women who had undergone labiaplasty in their study "tended to compare their own labial appearance with images they considered to be more valid representations. This was primarily the 'before' labiaplasty photographs on surgeons' websites." [One participant said:] "I'd seen a lot on the internet like lots of 'before' ones [photos] … I thought, oh my god, all these women are getting it [labiaplasty] done. Mine was still worse than theirs" [26]. A study by Howarth et al. found that "All participants identified a photograph of hairless female genitals with no visible labia minora as the societal 'ideal'" [25].
[6] This reason was given by a respondent to the Nuffield Council on Bioethics Online Questionnaire [27, p. 8]. Some researchers report that physical reasons for FGCS are given as a way of disguising the fact that the primary motivation is cosmetic [26].

[7] All these reasons were cited by respondents to the Nuffield Council on Bioethics Working Party on Cosmetic Procedures call for evidence [9].

Moreover, because FGCS applies only to women, it reinforces gender inequality more generally. Cosmetic surgery on men's genitals is far less common; many of the major commercial cosmetic surgery providers do not offer it. The fact that many women use images from pornography to identify the 'ideal' vulva also connects that ideal to the idea that women's bodies are primarily for the sexual satisfaction of men and should be appraised as a thing to be looked at by others rather than experienced from within.

FGCS is a procedure that can be chosen. But because the choice to undergo FGCS is affected by both the disadvantage and influence factors, it is a choice that should be questioned. The mere fact of choice is not enough to exonerate FGCS.

Policy Implications

Choices that are affected by the influence and disadvantage factors are unjust. Remedying that injustice can take several forms. It can involve reducing the costs of the practice, so that it no longer brings disadvantage. It can involve reducing the influence to undergo the practice, so that it can more honestly be described as an autonomous choice. It can involve regulating, restricting, or even banning the practice, so that it may not be chosen. These different methods can also be employed in combination.

Which option is best suited to FGCS? The disadvantage resulting from the practice is of three kinds: physical, financial and psychosocial. The physical costs of FGCS cannot easily be reduced. Reputable cosmetic surgeons should already be practising safely and professionally, striving to provide the best possible clinical outcome. The commercial cosmetic surgery industry is plagued with poor practice and inadequate regulation and there is room for improvement, but little government appetite for reform [9]. But no matter how skilled the surgeon, FGCS necessarily involves the removal of sensitive, healthy tissue, and brings risks of side effects and complications.

Attempting to solve the problem by reducing the financial costs is not promising. There is no commercial incentive to make the procedure cheaper, and provision on the NHS would normalise the procedure further while taking resources from other areas. And normalising the procedure means increasing the psychosocial costs, in the sense of entrenching the idea that many women have abnormal labia that should be corrected surgically.

The more promising strategy is thus to reduce the pressure to undergo FGCS. This can be done in a variety of ways involving a variety of actors. It can include education in schools and elsewhere – for girls and for boys – about the normal variety of bodily anatomy. It can involve educational programmes that seek to raise girls' and women's self-esteem and body confidence, and to reduce appearance-related anxiety. It can involve media, marketing, and advertising changes, either voluntarily or through regulators. The report *Cosmetic Procedures: Ethical Issues* contains many recommendations for reducing the pressures that lead women to demand cosmetic procedures of all kinds, and these apply to FGCS too [9].

What of legal measures that tackle the practice directly? The most obvious and simple legal move would be for the UK government to enforce the provisions of the UK Female Genital Mutilation Act 2003 and prosecute those who perform FGCS when it is not necessary for the patient's physical or mental health. This measure would have the advantage of restricting provision of FGCS but the disadvantage of encouraging both patients and practitioners to think of their natural labia as causing serious distress. Instead, then, the guidance notes of the legislation should be revised so that they no longer include the asymmetry between FGM sought for 'cultural' reasons and that sought for cosmetic reasons. As cosmetic considerations just are cultural considerations, there is no philosophical basis for this distinction [28], and it renders the law racist by effectively outlawing a practice for women from FGM-practising communities but not others.

This move, interpreting the Act as ruling out both FGM and FGCS, was in fact the intention of Parliamentarians. For example, Baroness Rendell said in the House of Lords in 2003:

> When the 1985 Act was passed, it was not Parliament's intention to place any statutory limitation on operations that are genuinely necessary; nor is it the intention of the Bill. Such operations may well be rare, but they do occur, and it would be wrong to criminalise them. But unless they are medically necessary, any operations involving mutilation of the external genitalia—"designer vagina" or otherwise—are already illegal if carried out by a person in the UK. Under the Bill's provisions, they will also be illegal if carried out by a UK national or permanent UK resident outside the UK. That will be the case even if the woman on whom the operation is carried out consents. [29]

In the House of Commons debate Sandra Gidley MP made a similar point, and also pointed to the dangers of racism:

> That observation brings me to an important point, because my understanding of the Bill is that it will make cosmetic surgery to the vaginal area illegal. I have no problem with that, but the issue should definitely be explored in Committee. It is regarded as a choice issue. I do not think that we should make any exceptions for white women expressing a choice for fashion reasons, when we are stopping black women, who may have no choice, perhaps because they are children, from having surgery. We must ensure that no distinction is drawn between these two practices, and it should all be part of the same message. [30]

One issue raised by my analysis is whether FGCS is distinct from other forms of cosmetic surgery. In many ways it is not. All cosmetic surgery takes place in a social context, one that is highly gendered and that encourages women in particular to place a high value on their appearance. There is an epidemic of appearance-related anxiety among young people and particularly young women [31], and all cosmetic surgery both contributes towards that anxiety and is made popular by it [9]. There is reason, in other words, to be concerned about cosmetic procedures in general, to enact stronger regulation on the industry itself and to work to counter the emphasis on body image that is found in media of all sorts and exacerbated by social media, marketing and youth culture.

But FGCS does have some distinctive features. In general, cosmetic procedures are more commonly performed on women than on men, but cosmetic genital surgery is still largely a procedure for women only. For example, major commercial providers such as Harley Medical Group and MYA Cosmetic Surgery offer cosmetic surgery on female genitals but not male ones, despite there being no legal restrictions on male genital cosmetic surgery. Moreover, the rapid and recent rise in popularity of FGCS, and the fact that the female genitals are otherwise so private and seldom seen, suggests its association with deeply sexist norms, connected with pornography and the fashion for complete hair removal. Several researchers note that the 'ideal' vulva that labiaplasty creates resembles that of a prepubescent girl [19, 22]. Finally, its connections to FGM mean that a consistent approach to eradicating FGM must necessarily tackle FGCS as well.

I have argued elsewhere that there are grounds for much greater restrictions on cosmetic procedures in general. As a brief summary, there are grounds for regulating or even prohibiting those cosmetic procedures that are both seriously risky or harmful and strongly connected to sex inequality [6]. And there are grounds for restricting *all* cosmetic procedures performed on children [9]. Objections to FGCS are not, therefore, unique to it. Nonetheless, FGCS remains a clear case of a practice that cannot be exonerated merely by an appeal to individual choice.

References

1. Royal College of Obstetricians and Gynaecologists Ethics Committee. Ethical Opinion Paper: Ethical considerations in relation to female genital cosmetic surgery (FGCS), 2013.

2. MYA Cosmetic Surgery. Labiaplasty. Available from: www.mya.co.uk/labiaplasty/#dqD4VLXScbtZAKUk.97

3. The Surrey Park Clinic. Labial reduction. Available from: www.thesurreyparkclinic.co.uk/treatments/surgical-procedures-in-clinic/labial-reduction/?gclid=CM6_5frxodYCFcsW0wodp-sBhg

4. Medico Beauty and IVF. Labiaplasty. Available from: https://medicobeautyclinic.com/aesthetic-surgery/procedures/labiaplasty-labia-minora-reduction

5. Mill JS. *On liberty*. In *Utilitarianism, on liberty, considerations on representative government*. London: Everyman; 1994.

6. Chambers C. *Sex, culture, and justice: The limits of choice*. University Park, PA: Pennsylvania State University Press; 2008.

7. Barry B. *Culture and equality: An egalitarian critique of multiculturalism*. Cambridge: Polity Press; 2001.

8. Chambers C. Judging women: Twenty-five years further toward a feminist theory of the state. *Feminist Philos Q*. 2007;3(2.5). https://doi.org/10.5206/fpq/2017.2.5

9. Nuffield Council on Bioethics. *Cosmetic procedures: Ethical issues*. London: Nuffield Council on Bioethics; 2017.

10. MacCallum F, Widdows H. Altered images: Understanding the influence of unrealistic images and beauty aspirations. *Health Care Analysis*. 2016. doi 10.1007/s10728-016-0327-1.

11. O'Connor R. Designer vagina surgery could be as illegal as FGM, Theresa May warns. *The Independent* (10 December 2014). Available from: www.independent.co.uk/news/uk/politics/designer-vagina-surgery-could-be-as-illegal-as-fgm-theresa-may-warns-9915466.html

12. Mills & Reeve. Briefing: The Female Genital Mutilation Act and its relation to female genital cosmetic surgery

(October 2013). Available from: www.mills-reeve.com/files/Publication/e023b495-a726-4241-b4dc-5d607f22 d2f4/Presentation/PublicationAttachment/efa6e8e7-1 4e1-498d-9496-5fc0bde49384/FGMA_Oct13.pdf

13. Berer M. Labia reduction for non-therapeutic purposes vs. female genital mutilation: contradictions in law and practice in Britain. *Reprod Health Matters.* 2010;18 (35). Available from: www.thefreelibrary.com/Labia+r eduction+for+non-therapeutic+reasons+vs.+female+ genital…-a0236247700

14. Crown Prosecution Service. Female genital mutilation legal guidance. Available from: www.cps.gov.uk/legal/ d_to_g/female_genital_mutilation/#a01

15. Explanatory Note to UK Female Genital Mutilation Act 2003. Available from: www.legislation.gov.uk/ukp ga/2003/31/contents

16. Davis K. *Reshaping the female body: The dilemma of plastic surgery.* London: Routledge; 1995.

17. Sharp G, Tiggemann M, Mattiske J. Factors that influence the decision to undergo labiaplasty: Media, relationships, and psychological well-being. *Aesthet Surg J.* 2016;36(4):469–78.

18. McCartney J. Great Wall of Vagina. Fine Art Studios. Available from: www.greatwallofvagina.co.uk/home

19. Rogers RG. Most women who undergo labiaplasty have normal anatomy; we should not perform labiaplasty. *Am J Obstet Gynecol.* 2014;211(3):218–20.

20. Crouch N, Deans R, Michala L, Liao LM, Creighton S. Clinical characteristics of well women seeking labial reduction surgery: A prospective study. *BJOG. Int J Obstet Gynaecol.* 2011;118:1507–10.

21. Greenfield L. *Generation wealth.* London: Phaidon Press; 2017.

22. Schick VR, Rima BN, Calabrese SK. Evulvaluation: The portrayal of women's external genitalia and physique across time and the current Barbie doll ideals. *J Sex Res.* 2010;48(1):74–81.

23. Braun V. Female genital cosmetic surgery: A critical review of current knowledge and contemporary debates. *J Womens Health.* 2010;19(7):1393–407.

24. Moran C, Lee C. What's normal? Influencing women's perceptions of normal genitalia: An experiment involving exposure to modified and nonmodified images. *BJOG.* 2014;121.

25. Howarth C, Hayes J, Simonis M, Temple-Smith M. 'Everything's neatly tucked away': Young women's views on desirable vulval anatomy. *Cult Health Sex.* 2016;18 (12). Available from: www.ncbi .nlm.nih.gov/pubmed/?term=Everything's+neatly+ tucked+away

26. Sharp G, Mattiske J, Vale KI. Motivations, expectations, and experiences of labiaplasty: A qualitative study. *Aesthet Surg J.* 2016;36(8): 920–8.

27. Nuffield Council on Bioethics Online Questionnaire, as summarized at http://nuffieldbioethics.org/wp-con tent/uploads/Survey-Monkey-Questionnaire-analysis .pdf

28. Chambers C. *Normal bodies: Cultural, cosmetic, and clinical surgery.* MS.

29. Baroness Rendell of Babergh, speaking in the debate on the Female Genital Mutilation Bill in the House of Lords. Hansard HL Deb. 12 September 2003, Vol 652 cc635-53. Available from: http://hansard.millbanksys tems.com/lords/2003/sep/12/female-genital-mutila tion-bill

30. Sandra Gidley (Romsey), speaking in the debate on the Female Genital Mutilation Bill in the House of Commons. Hansard HC Deb. 21 March 2003, Vol 401 cc1188-208. Available from: http://hansard.millbank systems.com/commons/2003/mar/21/female-genital-mutilation-bill.

31. Rumsey N, Harcourt D (eds). *Oxford handbook of the psychology of appearance.* Oxford: Oxford University Press; 2012.

A Historical Analysis of Beliefs Supporting Female Genital Cosmetic Surgery

Hera Cook

Introduction

For female cosmetic genital surgery (FCGS) to become a viable practice, major changes had to take place in women's attitudes and practices. This chapter describes how the conditions emerged to make demand for FCGS possible among Anglo-American women and girls from the last third of the nineteenth century until the 2000s. Consideration is given to women's sexual beliefs and practices; the role of hygiene; the basis for competition between girls and women; and the images of genitals that were available to them.

Women's sexual response is complex and highly variable between individuals [1]. The female organs involved in sexual pleasure, reproduction and excretion are packed tightly into a small area, with major bodily processes overlapping and impacting upon the others. In addition, there is a fundamental, strongly positive interaction between emotions and these organs or body parts, which is central to sexual arousal. Societal attitudes to female sexuality remain deeply contradictory. Questions about embodied sexual response raised in the 1920s, such as whether the cervix is involved in sexual arousal, remain unanswered [2, 3]. Women's understanding of these processes has been shaped by the incorrect, or incomplete, existing knowledge, as well as by imposed ignorance and censorship.

Labiaplasty, or the cutting away of 'excess' tissue from the labia minora, has become an increasingly well-known operation since the late 1990s. Yet, the *Kinsey Report on Sexual Behavior in the Human Female* (1953) found that 84% of the 2,727 women interviewed who had ever masturbated did so using labial and/or clitoral techniques. Women reported stroking or rhythmically pulling their labia minora [1]. Conversely, when performing clitorectomies to prevent masturbation in mid-nineteenth century London, the surgeon Issac Baker Brown brutally excised the labia [4, 5]. Why are women today, who say they want to improve their sexual experience, paying to have sexually responsive tissue removed? Surgeons who undertake labiaplasties argue that removal of labial tissue does not reduce sensitivity and, according to their research, women's sexual response is improved following the operation. Once the tissue is sliced off, it has, obviously, no sensitivity, so their claim must be that labia do not contribute to sexual response [6]. Kinsey et al. found that:

> Both the outer and the inner surfaces of the labia minora ... are highly sensitive to tactile stimulation ... As sources of erotic arousal, the labia minora seem to be fully as important as the clitoris ... During coitus, the entrance of the penis may provide considerable stimulation for the labia minora ... [at the lower end,] the labia minora continue inward to form a broad, funnel-shaped vestibule which leads to the ... introitus ... of the vagina [and is] as important a source of erotic stimulation as the labia minora or the clitoris [1].

The labia minora also react strongly during sexual arousal. They are highly innervated along the edge and sexual arousal leads them to engorge and double or triple in thickness, then change colour from pink to intense red when orgasm is imminent [7,8]. Yet it appears some women feel slicing away the labia minora improves sexual satisfaction. These claims about positive outcomes indicate that even the mere awareness that her genitals may be seen at by an other can destroy a woman's fragile, conscious connection with her embodied sexual response.

Socialisation and the Possible Causes of Change

The availability of images depicting standardised genitals, combined with advertising and media coverage of cosmetic surgery from the late 1990s, is frequently offered as the cause of women's rejection of their labia minora. Presentation of images cannot, however, in itself be held accountable for the acceptance of one look as ideal, or the rejection of another. The

acceptance of pubic hair removal, also proposed as a causal influence, is subject to the same caveat. Why has a particular genital look lent itself at this particular moment to being broadcast to a wider audience? Why has that audience responded with such anxiety about their own genitals that they are willing to remove sexually responsive tissue? Readiness to accept new practices and aesthetic standards is socially and culturally constructed.

Having FCGS is often understood as simply a choice made by an individual, but the feelings and attitudes that result in such choices are created by powerful social forces. Social construction refers to the shaping of people from infancy by their environment, which includes available resources, such as housing and food, as well as patterns of nurture and all other behaviour by people around the child. By far the larger part of socialisation is non-verbal learning, involving embodied knowledge and practices. Bodies, as well as beliefs and attitudes, are socially constructed [3, 9]. For example, a child growing up in the 1890s sharing a bedroom, or even a bed, in a home with no bathroom or indoor toilet would have found using the toilet more of an effort [10]. She might have been scared to go outside at night and discouraged from disturbing her siblings. Her capacity for sphincter control would probably have been greater than that of a child who grows up today sleeping in her own bedroom, possibly with an ensuite bathroom, and getting up to use the toilet whenever the urge strikes. As adults, however, both would have interpreted their feeling of a need to urinate as a response to a natural embodied demand which was/is independent of social or economic factors. Most people similarly experience their feelings of, and about, being sexually aroused as natural. This leaves a woman with no defence against the belief that there is something wrong with her if her genitals appear to look or respond differently to the way in which she believes those of other women look and respond.

The word culture refers to the systems of ideas existing and continually being developed in a society, which are evident in print media, including advertising, and in material objects. Cultural construction refers to shaping of beliefs and values. Subjectivity, a person's perspective and understanding, are shaped by cultural beliefs that, for example, bodily processes just happen 'naturally'; the person cannot not be aware of these beliefs and cannot not respond even if the response is to ignore, or reject, the accepted beliefs. As new circumstances emerge, people respond and, by doing so, create new ideas and practices from within the socio-economic relationships and culture they have inherited. When the object of concern is not openly discussed, as with genitals, the relationship between changing cultural beliefs and new emotional attitudes will often be obscure and confusing.

The concept of norms is central to understanding why women are vulnerable to the belief that their genitals require surgery to look acceptable and/or to improve their sexual response. Norms emerge in response to cultural beliefs about a given, regularly occurring action or state, such as frequency of urination, or sexual response. Individuals are sanctioned by society when they do not conform. Internalisation of norms causes individuals to conform by creating subjective beliefs in the necessity for the specified action, or persons may conform because they are avoiding sanctions. Norms evolve as practices are created based on existing values. Removal of body hair is an example of such development. Historically, the amount of hair on the face and easily visible body parts was subject to norms establishing whether a person was male or female. Those with too little or too little much hair in the correct places were vulnerable to taunting, such as a woman who grew a beard, or a man who could not. Once it became practical to remove face and body hair, the existence of those norms created a rationale supporting continuously increasing aspirations for a more female, that is, less hairy, body. The existence of alternatives, within subcultures or among other ethnic groups, may undermine norms, especially when the costs of compliance with the existing norms are increasing [11]. Thus socialisation establishes people's emotional and behavioural responses to their genitals; the individual's culturally constructed beliefs provide explanations for these responses; and norms shape how the responses are expressed.

Feeling and Touching: Fertility Control, Sexuality and Hygiene in the Early to Mid-Twentieth Century

Feeling and Touching the Body as a Source of Knowledge

Around 1900, around three-quarters of the British and US population were working class. Most of these women never saw their own naked bodies. Even small mirrors were luxuries, and most lived in crowded homes, with no running water, indoor toilets or separate bathrooms. Growing respectability discouraged girls from activities such as communal swimming, which were, anyway, less usual in cities. They rarely undressed fully and they experienced their bodies by feeling, rather than by looking. Historians have described how the full range of the senses, feeling/touching, hearing, tasting and smelling, were replaced as modes of perception by visual modes of seeing and learning in the sixteenth and seventeenth centuries [12]. Demands for female modesty and sexual reticence placed respectable female sexuality outside this trajectory. Despite the rise in literacy by the late nineteenth century, girls in all classes continued to learn about their genitals and sexuality/reproduction through feeling and touching [10, 13]. Mothers in this period were often too inhibited to talk about sexuality and reproductive processes [10, 14]. The distress ensuing from the resulting ignorance could be substantial [3]: potential advantages to this culture of touch and feeling rather than seeing lay in the potential for the private discovery of personal sexual sensations and emotions [1].

Sexuality and Fertility Control

In the early nineteenth century, fertility rates were historically high and the existing methods of birth control and abortion were either not effective or posed risks to health [3]. Effective approaches to preventing births severely limited sexual activity; delaying marriage (including sexual intercourse), followed by marital restraint or even abstinence from sexual intercourse once married [3, 15, 16]. The burden of embodied reproductive labour that high fertility imposed on women gave them a stronger motivation to forgo sexual pleasure than the solely economic pressure men shared with their wives [3]. In achieving the required control, women and some men developed an almost abstract fear of embodied sexual desire, producing a culture of prudish respectability that peaked around 1900 (not during the so-called Victorian era of the mid-nineteenth century) and was probably stronger in Britain than in other European cultures or in the United States [3, 17]. For many, if not most, women in the late nineteenth century, particularly in Britain, disgust was more prominent than pleasure as the normal response to evidence of embodied sexuality, including the genitals of both sexes. This emotion serves to defend the self against psychological and physical contamination

and reflected the belief that sexuality was powerfully polluting. The belief that masturbation caused a wide variety of diseases emerged in the eighteenth century and, though this fear peaked around 1900, these anxieties continued to strongly reinforce negative feelings about the genitals, dwindling into strong embarrassment, or defiant promotion, only in the last third of the twentieth century [3, 18].

Research into British pornography found that around 1880, 'eroticism in some fundamental way became equivalent with dirtiness' [19]. In the United States sexual repression seems to have been less extreme and dominant than in Britain, but anxieties about hygiene appear to have been greater. Scientific discoveries emphasised the association of 'dirt' with disease and this fused with anxieties about sexuality, reinforced by high rates of syphilis [20]. For most women their genitals were a dirty part of the body to avoid and think about as little as possible. Being seen to be dirty was increasingly shameful, lower class and might expose a person to taunts and to being seen as ugly. Engaging in more demanding and not yet fully established hygiene practices was, on the other hand, innovative and modern. It established status, gave righteousness and was seen as more beautiful. Even when aspirations are new, congruence with such associations and beliefs built up over decades and centuries makes pressure for conformity to norms very difficult to resist.

Cultural Knowledge and Women's Awareness of Their Sexual/Reproductive Organs

In the late nineteenth century, the majority of women were ignorant even of the existing knowledge about their sexual and reproductive organs and processes. Cultural radicals believed that provision of sexual knowledge, which came to be termed sex education, would improve women's well-being. The response of Marie Bonaparte, a wealthy French psychoanalyst, reveals that the emerging 'knowledge' about women's sexual response failed to provide simple answers. Sigmund Freud's developmental theory shaped cultural beliefs about female sexual response in the first two-thirds of the twentieth century; he argued a girl's sexual feeling began in infancy with clitoral (masturbatory) sensations which were independent and masculine. Maturity involved the transfer of her erotic response to the vagina and the achievement of feminine orgasms in coitus. Freud's belief that female sexual response should be confined to vaginal intercourse was widely shared but the importance he placed on infantile masturbation and the child's sexual feelings was extremely challenging.

Bonaparte was tormented by her frigidity, defined as the failure to have mature vaginal orgasms in coitus [21, 22]. She collected data on other women and concluded this failure could be caused by too great a distance between the clitoris and the vagina. An Austrian surgeon, Josef Halban, created a procedure in which the suspensory ligament of the clitoris was transected and the clitoral glans was moved downward, closer to the vaginal entrance [23]. To achieve this, the surgery had to slice the clitoris away from the underlying and surrounding structures. Anatomical knowledge of clitoral anatomy revealing the destruction the operation would cause was available [24]. Bonaparte did not value clitoral sensation because she was convinced neuroses and unhappiness were produced by women's reliance on masculine clitoral sensation. Halban performed the operation on Bonaparte three times, in 1927, 1930 and 1931, before they decided surgical approach was misconceived. That such an intelligent woman should have gone down this route illustrates the distress that feelings of sexual inadequacy and unfulfilled desire produced in response to sexual and gender norms.

Ignorance and anxiety could cause very different problems. Vaginismus, which is the unconscious clamping of the vaginal muscles such that the penis cannot enter (without force) and intercourse take place, was an extreme response of some women to fears about sexuality and giving birth. In 1958, a three-year training seminar was held in London on treatment of non-consummated marriages, during which the participating doctors saw around 700 cases, in many of which the woman experienced vaginismus [25]. Treatment involved talking with the patient and then insertion of glass dilators into her vagina to encourage acceptance that the penis would not cause damage; feelings of disgust led to worse outcomes than fear and anxiety. These women's unconscious use of their vaginal muscles highlights the extent to which their socialisation had resulted in an absence of capacity for conscious use of their genital musculature.

Vaginismus still occurs today, though these feelings are far less usual. Fear about the impact of giving birth may, however, have grown. Birth may result in

some changes to the vagina ranging from imperceptible to significant; only a small proportion of women require surgical repair. In some Asian cultures, strippers perform a show that consists of women using their pelvic muscles to hold in, or eject over a distance from their vagina objects such as ping pong balls. Leaving aside the exploitation involved, this act reveals a radically different cultural awareness of the vagina. The strippers' act would have been inconceivable to Western women, who overwhelmingly were unaware their vaginas had any muscles, or that these muscles could play a role in protecting their vagina during childbirth and in increasing sexual pleasure. Kinsey et al. found that deep insertion of objects into the vagina by early to mid-twentieth century US women during masturbation was almost unheard of and even shallow insertion of fingers was rare, showing their socialisation resulted in a lack of awareness of potential pleasure [1]. Embodied experience produced through socialisation contributes in such instances to poorer outcomes for women.

Starting to Look at Female Bodies, Advertisers, Birth Control and Cultural Radicals

Advertisers Appropriating Feminism to Sell New Products, Including Birth Control

US advertisers appropriated feminist rhetoric in the 1920s, representing modern emancipated women as exercising their new agency by choosing between alternative products. Following World War I, there had been a huge growth in women's confidence. In 1918, English women aged over thirty were given the vote, and all US women were guaranteed the right to vote in 1920 by the Nineteenth Amendment. Even at the peak of the struggle for women's suffrage, relatively few women were active feminists; but, following World War I, what had been radical ideas about women's capacity and their right to make choices about their lives became commonsense for the younger generation. Young American women in the 1920s connected female heterosexual expression with defiance and pleasure, while feminism was, largely correctly, associated with the sexually repressive Victorian sensibilities of older women. The radical feminists of the 1910s, or the earlier free lovers, radicals and sex hygienists, had been few in number and their ideas received little attention [24]. Young women rejected female submissiveness and sacrifice to duty but few aspired to higher education or careers, most had little education or political awareness and minimal exposure to feminist ideas. The consumption of attractive new products, often purporting to be supported by medical or scientific authorities, was compatible with their aspirations [25]. Many of these products required considerable further development or were expensive, including toothpastes, deodorants, sanitary pads, shampoo and safety razors. Nonetheless, in this period, young women began to interpret their body as a project, which they could use products to improve and develop [26, 27].

Rising product consumption and feminism created the context in which Anglo-American women began to use products in their vaginas. US advertisers spent very heavily promoting Lysol® and other douches as 'feminine hygiene' products, a covert means of referring to birth control [25]. By 1930, 60% of white married US couples were limiting their fertility but most were doing so with male-controlled methods such as condoms and, especially, withdrawal, which involved no commercial products. By 1940, antiseptic vaginal douches were the most widely used method by US women in all classes [25]. In the 1950s, more than two-thirds of US women (68%) used methods that required them to insert items, including diaphragms and douches, into their vaginas, compared to under a quarter of British women (24.5%) [28, 29]. British women were less willing to touch their genitals and both British men and women were uncomfortable with women being seen to initiate sex by inserting birth control devices before intercourse [3]. In this context, their reticence had advantages; commercial douches such as Lysol® were caustic disinfectants, also used for cleaning the home, which caused injury, and even deaths, when not properly diluted [25].

Existing beliefs primed women to accept that strong disinfectants were required to make the vagina 'clean'. There has been considerable historical research on such advertising [14, 24, 25, 27] in the United States but little on the topic in the United Kingdom. It is probable there was less advertising of intimate products, as the British were less affluent, more sexually reticent and more resistant to intrusive internal practices [3]. Even so, a British medical textbook gave an example of a 'young woman in her twenties [who] presented with a severe vaginal and vulval condition as the result of douching four times

daily with Lysol, in an excess of zeal for cleanliness' [30]. In this period, desire for control of fertility encouraged US women to accept the authority of advertisers and to disregard discomfort caused by the products, while for many British women, control over fertility continued to be achieved by male domination of sexual practice and comparatively less experience of sexual pleasure [3].

Seeing Naked Bodies

Norms around the look of the vulval area did not exist in the interwar period. The response of the cultural radicals in the early Anglo-American Nudist movement to naked bodies highlights the lack of familiarity and ambivalence with which naked bodies were viewed even by those disposed to reject existing inhibitions [31]. In the late 1920s, radical nudists had claimed that 'the widespread practice of nudism would … restore the body to the importance and dignity to which it is entitled' [32]. When they were faced with large numbers of actual bodies, however, these people found them ugly. This response occurs throughout the writing on nudism. Maurice Parmelee, a US sociologist, devoted a chapter of his book *Nudism in Modern Life* to analysing the body part by part. Comments included: "To anyone who has an ideal of a beautifully formed body, the feet are blots and eyesores … the most frequent and hideous cases are among the women ... The abdomen is the ugliest portion of the human form in a vast number of individuals probably the majority of mankind"[32]. Cultural expectations of naked bodies were based on classical Greek and Roman statues: white and smooth, firm and hairless.

Parmelee explained that his prescriptions for male and female beauty were based on such "statues as the Aphrodite of Melo … generally regarded as beautiful because they confirm [sic] or are supposed to confirm to the 'perfect' that is to say normal human type". Confusion of the ideal and the norm is central to the compulsion that norms about bodies produce. Equating being normal with meeting the (rising) ideal creates constant pressure to improve. Within the classical framework, nakedness was idealised as heroic and divine, associated with whiteness and civilisation [33]. The nudists' shock when faced with living bodies reveals the absence of a positive cultural framework in which to situate even the genitals of white women, while those of other ethnicities were excluded *de facto*. In 2002, cultural critic Simone Weil Davis described labia minora as 'gateway' tissue, which is 'somewhat indeterminate in texture and hue, yielding slowly from outer to inner and blurring the boundary between the fetishized gloss of the outer dermis and the wet mushy darkness of the inside' [34]. This lack of clear definition of boundaries, form and colour is contrary to classical/modern beauty criteria. Female genitals are experienced by heterosexual men as sexually arousing but there was no existing cultural framework within which women, especially, could construct genitals as visually beautiful.

Constructing New Genital Norms Looking and Seeing Women's Vulvas

Genitals in Men's Magazines and in the Women's Liberation Movement

Women had no image of a norm/ideal against which to compare and assess the attractiveness of their own genitals even if the desire to do so had occurred to them. Prior to World War I, genital norms appear to have been limited to the expectation that the body would conform to the binary division into male and female, with appropriate genitalia [35]. Explicit photographs of sexual acts showing a wide variety of female genitals and bodies with body hair were produced from the mid-nineteenth century but these were sold covertly to men [36]. They were not available legally, nor would they have been acceptable to the vast majority of respectable women. From the 1950s, naked female breasts and semi-exposed bodies were visible in the nudist magazines and in the new mainstream men's magazines. Many children found sex manuals hidden in their parents' bedrooms and, by the late 1960s, diagrams and occasionally even photographs of genitals were also included in the sex education books culturally radical parents bought for their children. *Playboy* centerfolds have attracted researchers but the earliest claimed appearance of pubic hair was in *Penthouse* in 1970, while *Hustler* published the first "pink shots" of labial flesh in 1974 [37]. Explicit images of genitals remained the province of illegal pornography.

Meanwhile, small groups in the Women's Liberation Movement (WLM) had been encouraging women to use a mirror and, if they had access to one, a vaginal speculum, to look at, and into, their own genitals. The Boston Women's Health Collective wrote *Our Bodies, Ourselves* and began sharing genital self-examination with a larger audience in 1970. To everyone's surprise, the book sold 250,000 copies in the first year. By 1976, the commercial edition had sold 2.5 million but *Playboy* alone sold 5.6 million copies in 1975 [38]. Both the women's health movement and men's magazines faced down censorship and contributed to the new openness and the 'right to know' politically and socially [39]. But the WLM consisted of a small number of anti-capitalist young women with no resources other than collective commitment and ideas that spoke to their audience, whereas mainstream men's magazines were part of a well-capitalised, high-profit industry. It is difficult to underestimate the importance of the limited resources available for spreading new ideas that were not consistent with advertising messages or mainstream institutions. Nonetheless, and despite the way in which, as with first wave feminism in the 1920s, WLM ideas were co-opted and distorted for audiences that had no contact with the originals, the WLM did establish an enduring discourse in opposition to the advertising/medicine /hygiene construction of the woman's body as a project, which she was responsible for maintaining and improving in accordance with societal demands.

Arguably, this happened largely despite WLM socialists who believed that personal life was a distraction from anti-capitalist politics. Even *Our Bodies, Ourselves* had nothing to say about shaving legs or wearing make-up but in the photo of the woman examining her genitals, the spectator can see she has hairy legs [40]. Rejecting the capitalist, consumption-oriented construction of femininity was part of how those in the WLM lived. They were part of the counterculture, which had descended from the cultural radicals. The hippies' conception of a natural body and way of living that included allowing body hair to grow, wearing loose clothing, and bare feet, was influential, as were lesbians and, conversely, feminists who insisted that the pleasure women find in clothing, and in decorating and adorning their bodies could not be reduced to consumption and competition for men. Wearing second-hand clothing was one form of resistance. In 1970, Australian, anarcho-feminist Germaine Greer fiercely rejected vaginal deodorants and the claim that female genitals smell, and suggested instead that women should taste their own menstrual blood [41]. Feminist artists and activists began production of an ongoing stream of genitally focused art works, including Judy Chicago's 'The Dinner Party,' which is uniquely celebratory of the vulva. The work consists of a three-sided table with individualised place settings for fifty famous women, on which are plates with highly coloured stylised labia in deep, fleshy relief [42]. By the late 1980s, there was a new awareness of looking at women's genitals across a wide spectrum of the culture.

Competition and Ranking of the Self among and by Women

Conventional Feminism and Competition between Women

Second-wave feminism rapidly became a broader movement, led by women with aspirations to succeed in the existing man's world, not to change society. This conventional feminism was powered by the competitiveness that women have internalised over the past century. Historically, within local communities competition between young women had played a limited, albeit important, role in their lives. Monogamous marriages broken by the death of a spouse were the norm, and a women's status as a wife, mother and housekeeper was stable and enduring. The deciding event in most women's lives was if, and who, they married. Cultural norms of beauty, while important, were little more than loosely defined archetypes. Young, unmarried women were potentially competing with other women for husbands; they were not competing with men. And they compared themselves with other women when deciding what was desirable in a woman, not with men. Women's comparison of themselves with other women helped drive the development of body norms and ideals.

From the late nineteenth century, formal education began to socialise children to accept a world in which formal ranking of self against others was routine; meeting external, non-familial standards from outside the immediate community started to become part of the lives of girls and young women. From the 1920s, women's magazines presented exhortations to improve and excel at the business of being a woman [43]. Individual achievement and self-determination, as well as emotional control, were presented as central to the cult of femininity. In the same decades, girls were increasingly told that they could succeed in education and get a higher status, thus expanding the arena of competition. Most occupations were still sex segregated and in the workplace, as in the home and local community, women were competing with other women.

In the 1950s, experts and advertisers began insisting that maintaining the female body was not just for the young; it was a life-long project necessary to the sexual success of a woman's marriage and in turn to ensuring her husband's faithfulness. Wives had to prevent themselves from becoming 'fat, shapeless' or 'scrawny', or marital unhappiness and divorce would result [44]. Body modifications, initially dieting, and then exercise, as well as use of cosmetics, were strongly promoted. The products introduced in the interwar period became affordable and their quality improved. Some met important needs: toothpaste improved dental health and menstrual products made women's lives easier. In contrast, removal by women of hair felt to be excessive began in the United States with the introduction of safety razors during the interwar period; these made self-removal of body hair in private practical; hairless legs quickly became a norm. Since the 1920s, advertisers have sold products and grooming as independent, self-care activities but concepts such as 'because you're worth it' derive from the rise of individualism and conventional, self-oriented feminism, not from activist feminism. This emphasises joining together with other women to improve conditions for women and is based on a larger vision than the betterment of the individual or her kin.

In the 1950s, marriages endured for longer than ever before due to improved mortality rates but by the 1970s, illegitimacy and divorce rates were rising sharply and casual sex and serial relationships were becoming more acceptable for young women. This meant that instead of a brief period of courting in which women assessed themselves and their looks against other women, or even the labour of keeping a husband faithful, competition for partners between sexually active women could be a lifelong project.

Sexual Practice; Looking and Being Seen

During the 1960s, oral contraception, or the Pill, radically transformed sexual mores, giving women almost complete control over their fertility [45]. Particularly among young unmarried people, however, the separation of sex and reproduction also resulted in sexual practice more closely focused on sexual intercourse, as there was no longer a need for 'petting' to avoid intercourse and the risk of pregnancy. Accounts of young unmarried people petting, that is fondling each other's bodies go back for centuries [46]. Lengthy mutual petting, like masturbation, had developed women's (and men's) awareness of their body's sexual response. The shift away from petting was an important aspect of the substantial shift taking place away from a woman's genitals being a source of sensation known by touch, to a body part that is looked at and possibly judged by others. This change was reinforced by affluence, which enabled young unmarried people to live separately from their parents, enabling more relaxed sexual activity and opportunities to look at each other's bodies.

No evidence has appeared in my research suggesting men had any appetite for doctored female genitals, or indeed for hairless pubes, though they have been willing to accept, and then insist on, the results of innovation [3]. Where a new trend was established by desirable and high-status women (according to whatever criteria), men would then incorporate this into their conception of the female norm. Surveys show numbers of sexual partners rising sharply into the early 2000s. Historically, the dominant role of the male in sexual activity was a given, but pleasurable sexual activity had also been strongly associated with privacy, trust and intimate emotion, especially for women [3]. A high turnover of partners means trust and getting to know each other are no longer so central to sexual activity, and the female body is experienced as an object to be looked at by the other, rather than as a source of feelings and sensations of touch while fondling in the dark.

Genital piercing was a socially challenging form of decoration initially taken up in the late 1980s by young women who rejected conventional femininity and, often, conventional feminism. Some among the older generation of women believed decoration of the genitals transgressed natural divisions of private and public but genital piercing was rather a sign that these divisions had broken down in young women's lives [47]. Acceptance by women from the late 1990s of the removal of their traditionally erotically arousing pubic hair may also in part reflect the new construction of the genitals as semi-public body parts. Hair removal was, however, also a central component of the trajectory of increasing body work [48]. By the 1990s, a context existed of constant work on head hair, including eyebrows and the normalisation of dyeing grey hair, and the removal of hair from all other parts of the body. The white, higher income women whose bodies conform most easily to the classical beauty ideal, and who took the lead in removing pubic hair, are also taking the lead in FCGS [49].

Conclusion

Twentieth-century women inherited powerful negative attitudes towards the body parts involved in sexuality, excretion and reproduction. In the first two-thirds of the century, new products transformed women's experience of their bodies, including their genitals, but with this came advertising that co-opted feminism and the new pleasure provided by baths and running hot and cold water to market damaging and ineffective products. Meanwhile, women were learning to compete in every area of their lives, not just while courting, and the body was becoming a project into which they poured effort. Women's experience of sexual pleasure is entwined with their capacity to control their fertility (including having wanted babies). Over the past two centuries, women and men have engaged in a process of experimentation with contraceptive methods that has reshaped heterosexual sexual activity [3]. The sexual culture of the young has largely moved from repressive insistence on the sexual ignorance of young women towards a performance-oriented, semi-public activity that leaves sexually active young women exposed to male judgement. FCGS operations are taking place in a small and crowded section of the female body on highly complex organs and tissue. Female sexual response involves mind–emotion–body interactions about which researchers and surgeons still know very little, and which are usually beyond the conscious control of the woman. In the supposed cause of improving women's sexual function by making them feel better, surgeons are scarring and destroying sexually responsive tissue. There has been development of a multifaceted discourse, rejecting the sexual and hygienic rationales for a further extension of prescriptive body norms to include the genitals. There is hope that women will reject the chewed up stumps left when surgeons have finished slicing and stitching away at their labia minora, and other mutilating operations, and learn to take a new delight in their own colorful, luscious, delicious and sexually responsive genitalia.

References

1. Kinsey AC, Pomeroy WB, Martin CE, Gebhard PH. *Sexual behavior in the human female*. Philadelphia: W. B. Saunders; 1953.

2. Levin RL. The involvement of the human cervix in reproduction and sex. *Sex Relat Ther.* 2005;20:251–60.

3. Cook H. *The long sexual revolution: English women, sex and contraception, 1800–1975.* Oxford: Oxford University Press; 2004.

4. *BMJ*, April 6, 1867, 407–8.

5. Scull A, Favreau D. The clitoridectomy craze. *Soc Res.* 1986;53:243–60.

6. Goodman MP. *Female genital plastic and cosmetic surgery.* Chichester: Wiley; 2016.

7. Dickinson RL. *Atlas of human sex anatomy.* 2nd ed. Baltimore: Williams & Wilkins; 1949.

8. Masters W, Johnson VE. *Human sexual response.* Boston, MA: Little Brown; 1966.

9. Fausto-Sterling A. The bare bones of sex: Part 1 – Sex and gender. *Signs.* 2005; 30(2): 1491–1527.

10. Cook H. Emotion, bodies, sexuality, and sex education in Edwardian England. *Histor J.* 2012; 55(2): 475–95.

11. Horne C. Sociological perspectives on the emergence of norms. In Hechter M, Opp K (eds), *Social norms.* New York: Russell Sage Foundation; 2001, pp. 3–33.

12. Corbin A. Charting the cultural history of the senses. In Howes D (ed), *Empire of the senses: The sensual culture reader.* Oxford: Berg; 2005.

13. Reagan LJ. *When abortion was a crime: Women, medicine, and law in the United States, 1867–1973.* Berkeley: University of California Press; 1997.

14. Klean Zwilling JM. *Euphemistic rhetoric in advertising during the Comstock era: The importance of persona and cultural context in the Lysol case.* Unpublished PhD thesis, University of Illinois at Urbana-Champaign, 2017.

15. David PA, Sanderson WC. Rudimentary contraceptive methods and the American transition to marital fertility control, 1855–1915. In Engerman SL, Gallman RE (eds), *Long term factors in America's economic growth.* Chicago: University of Chicago Press; 1986, pp. 346–7.

16. Szreter S. *Fertility, class and gender in Britain, 1860–1940.* Cambridge: Cambridge University Press; 1996.

17. Freedman EB, D'Emilio J. *Intimate matters: A history of sexuality in America.* New York: Harper and Row; 1988.

18. Hare EH. Masturbatory insanity: The history of an idea. *J Ment Sci.* 1962;108:1–25.

19. Sigel LZ. Name your pleasure: The transformation of sexual language in nineteenth-century British pornography. *J Hist Sex* 2000;9:395–419.

20. Tomes N. The private side of public health: Sanitary science, domestic hygiene, and the germ theory, 1870–1900. *Bull Hist Med.* 1990;64:509–39.

21. Bertin C. *Marie Bonaparte: A life.* New York: Harcourt Brace Jovanovich; 1982.

22. Frederickson BF. Jomo Kenyatta, Marie Bonaparte and Bronislaw Malinowski on clitoridectomy and female sexuality. *Hist Workshop J.* 2008;65:23–48.

23. Bonaparte B. *Female sexuality.* London: Imago; 1953.

24. Cott NF. *The grounding of modern feminism.* New Haven, CT: Yale University Press; 1987.

25. Tone A. Contraceptive consumers: Gender and the political economy of birth control in the 1930s. *J Soc Hist.* 1996;29(3):485–506.

26. Vostral SL. Masking menstruation: The emergence of menstrual hygiene products in the United States. In Shail A, Howie G (eds), *Menstruation: A cultural history.* London: Palgrave Macmillan; 2005.

27. Marchand R. *Advertising the American dream: Making way for modernity, 1920–1940.* Berkeley: University of California Press; 1985.

28. Rowntree G, Pierce RM. Birth control in Britain: Part two. *Populat Stud* 1961;15:121–60.

29. Whelpton PK, Campbell AC, Freedman R. *Family planning, sterility and population growth.* New York: McGraw-Hill; 1959.

30. Hunt E. *Diseases affecting the vulva.* London: Henry Kimpton, 1943.

31. Cook H. Nudism: Sex, gender and social change, 1994. Unpublished paper. Available from the author upon request.

32. Parmelee M. *Nudism in modern life and the new gymnosophy.* London: Sunshine Book Company, 1933; revised edn, 1941.

33. Painter NI. *The history of white people.* New York: W. W. Norton; 2010.

34. Davis SW. Loose lips sink ships. *Feminist Stud.* 2002;28:7–35.

35. Mak G. *Doubting sex: Inscriptions, bodies and selves in nineteenth century hermaphrodite case histories.* Manchester: Manchester University Press; 2012.

36. Mirsky L, Rotenberg M. *The Rotenberg collection. Forbidden erotica.* Cologne: Taschen; 2000.

37. Kipnis L. *Bound and gagged pornography and the politics of fantasy in America.* Durham, NC: Duke University Press; 1999.

38. Davis K. *The making of* Our bodies, Ourselves: *How feminism travels across borders.* Durham, NC: Duke University Press; 2007.

39. Schudson M. *The rise of the right to know: Politics and the culture of transparency, 1945–1975.* Boston, MA: Harvard University Press; 2015.

40. Boston Women's Collective. *Our Bodies, Ourselves: A book by and for women*, New York: Simon and Schuster; 1973.

41. Greer G. *The female eunuch*: London: McGibbon & Kee; 1970.

42. www.judychicago.com/gallery/the-dinner-party/dp-artwork/

43. Ferguson M. *Forever feminine: Women's magazines and the cult of femininity*. London: Heinemann; 1983.

44. Zweiniger-Bargielowska I. *Women in 20th century Britain*. London: Longmans; 2001.

45. Cook H. The English sexual revolution: Technology and social change. *Hist Workshop J.* 2005;59:109–28.

46. Hitchcock T. Sociability and misogyny in the life of John Cannon, 1684–1743. In Hitchcock T, Cohen M (eds), *English masculinities, 1660–1800*. London: Longman; 1999.

47. Brumberg JJ. *The body project an intimate history of American girls*. New York: Random House; 1987.

48. Rowen TS, Thomas W, Gaither BS, et al. Pubic hair grooming prevalence and motivation among women in the United States. *JAMA Dermatol.* 2016;152:1106–113.

49. Cofield, L. *After shave: A cultural history of pubic hair removal in twentieth and twenty-first century Britain*. Forthcoming PhD, University of Sussex, 2018.

Feminist Activism to Challenge the New Industry of Female Genital Cosmetic Surgery

Leonore Tiefer

Introduction: From Critique to Activism

Feminists view activism as a complement to scholarship and journalism. Female genital cosmetic surgery (FGCS) scholarship names, analyzes, and deconstructs the various components of a new surgical industry managing women's bodies. As this book shows, recent scholarship has examined FCGS types, prevalence, justifications, proponents, and enabling factors. FGCS journalism tells individual stories of doctors and patients and offers accurate (sometimes) and misleading (too often) local information. FGCS activism attempts to disrupt the industry.

Many chapters in this book of interdisciplinary FGCS scholarship are likely to be critical of the industry while acknowledging the rights of individual surgery consumers. With any luck these chapters will lay out the scholarly landscape of FCGS: Who, What, When, Where, How, and, above all, Why.

But some of us coming from a feminist viewpoint who are critical of this new industry feel an urgency to go further and to take public action to diminish its impact, even to eradicate its existence. There is no recipe for such activism, or any activism, for that matter, no definitive list of successful or to-be-avoided strategies, and most of us who want to supplement our scholarship with activism are amateurs in the public realm. I came, for example, from a background in academic sex research and clinical sexology, and this chapter will offer my perspective on FGCS activism based on a decade's (2007–2017) efforts [1].

Professionals and Activism: Tension and Disincentive

Academics have often focused their scholarship on social problems and in recent decades have participated in many types of campus and community advocacy activities. Yet, there is an enduring "chasm" between activists and the academics who research and write about social issues and movements that bespeaks a "creative tension between thinking and action, between theory and practice" that limits academics' ability to engage in political activism (p. xii) [2].

Professional codes and traditions of conduct have likewise inhibited doctors, nurses, and lawyers from getting involved in social change activities. Professionals are encouraged to advocate for their clients and patients, but fear of jeopardizing their professional standing, licensure, or employment often discourages professionals' public advocacy behavior. Over five decades (1960s–2010s) as a sex educator and researcher, a licensed New York psychologist and sex therapist, and a member of many professional organizations, I saw very little attention paid to advocacy in scores of professional conferences – no workshops teaching activism skills, no plenaries describing successful activist campaigns, no lectures highlighting needed areas for advocacy. If activism was mentioned at all, it was informally, when conference attendees discussed their "private lives." I learned that activism was something some professionals did in their spare time, not as part of their career.

The exception to this was in feminist professional groups such as the Association for Women in Psychology or the Society for Menstrual Cycle Research, where politics was a regular topic of invited lectures and participatory workshops and where activist demonstrations were on occasion even scheduled into the program. Framing one's career in terms of "scholar-activism" was acceptable, even popular, in these groups, reflecting the goal of social change at the core of feminism.

Focus of the FGCS Activist Agenda: Reduce Both Demand and Supply

The FCGS industry is linked to numerous socioeconomic factors and agents as identified in other chapters in this book. Challenges require both short-term and long-term goals and utilization of a wide array of strategies and tactics. I see the FGCS activist agenda as a combination of campaigns to reduce both the demand for and the supply of FCGS insofar as the growth of the industry has come about because of increases in both. Success will require attacking both ends of the problem.

Reducing the demand for FGCS will be accomplished by increasing its negatives and decreasing its positives in the eyes of both consumers and professionals. By "increasing the negatives" I mean raising awareness of harmful consequences and side effects, increasing the financial cost, and stigmatizing consumers as gullible and professionals as exploitative. Raising awareness largely involves disseminating research, opinion pieces, and personal stories through teaching and speaking opportunities along with using commercial and social media.

"Decreasing the positives" of FGCS must also focus both on FCGS practitioners and the public and includes public education campaigns that highlight diverse untreated vulvas and their attractiveness, legal challenges to FGCS advertising, promoting restrictive professional guidelines for genital surgeries, and shaming FGCS practitioners. Obviously, activities such as "shaming" and "stigmatizing" are controversial and not for the faint of heart, but insofar as they are undertaken indirectly, these terms are not used. I thought it advisable, however, to be candid in this chapter about how activists construe their strategies.

The effectiveness of such activist efforts should be measured by demonstrating increasingly negative public attitudes toward FGCS and reduced FGCS availability and utilization. Documenting these types of changes is not easy, however. An ideal study would conduct a baseline survey prior to any action and then collect results on the same or a similar survey afterwards. While there have been a few FGCS attitude surveys, they are limited by the circumstances of collection, sample used, and questions asked [3], and I do not know of any repeated measures evaluating the effectiveness of FGCS activist campaigns. Future activism should consider incorporating before-and-after survey elements to document attitude changes.

Measuring the decline in FGCS utilization is also difficult. Journalism often presents statistics on the prevalence of FGCS procedures, from the American Society of Plastic Surgeons, for example [4], and articles in recent years have pointed to increasing numbers as a sign of the growing popularity of FGCS. However, methods of collecting such data and the clarity of classifications are confusing and controversial, and while we see many numbers floating around and lots more media attention to FGCS it is premature to conclude that prevalence is on the rise.

Examples of Campaigns Challenging FGCS

Activist projects focusing on FGCS vary greatly based on duration, style, focus, structure, and membership. Some involve direct action; some have a longer-term focus on changing public and professional attitudes. Some are stand-alone projects; some emerge from women's health or sexuality organizations. Some are one-person initiatives; some have large teams of participants. We know about most of them only because of media coverage. I would venture that college campus and women's health organization activist initiatives are numerous. As the media attention to FGCS grows, resistance also grows and activism becomes more salient and acceptable.

The largest group of activist projects I have identified are "vulva-positive" campaigns that celebrate the diversity of the vulva and explicitly accentuate its attractiveness. They aim to decrease the positives of FGCS by reducing genital disgust and dissatisfaction. In March, 2016, for example, I learned of a small sewing project in the United Kingdom. Julia Williams had been holding workshops to design patchwork vaginas out of fabric, fur, and glitter to promote body confidence and raise awareness of genital mutilation. "The artist and mum-of-two started the movement as a response to the growing trend for women to undergo labiaplasty or 'designer vagina' operations" [5]. I found out about this project accidentally online and believe there are many more. Here are some I have followed.

Great Wall of Vagina

In 2008, British sculptor Jamie McCartney made plaster casts of hundreds of women's vulvas, and created an artwork he called "The Great Wall of Vagina" [6]. Initially shocking, a decade later it is now clear that

McCartney's work was the beginning of a wave of vulva-positive art. The "Great Wall" has been widely exhibited and you can learn about a dozen spinoff projects on its website. A project called "Extremes" specifically speaks to FGCS activism:

EXTREMES – Another way to demonstrate human diversity is to concentrate on extremes or on certain themes. Thus we are also seeking women who fit into these categories: If you have particularly LARGE or SMALL LABIA or CLITORIS or you have anything you consider or know is UNUSUAL down there like multiple piercings, hypertrophia, hyperelasticity, childbirth changes etc and are willing to anonymously share it with the world then do get in touch. For many women, modeling for these works has been a real catharsis that alleviates personal anxieties. Once you cross that Rubicon you are free! *(capitals in the original)* [7]

V-Day

Playwright Eve Ensler wrote and performed a one-woman play called *The Vagina Monologues* in New York in 1996 [8]. Among other topics, this piece celebrated women's genitalia. Despite criticisms of some of its politics, it has continued to be hugely popular and performed on college campuses and in communities around the world. In 1998, Ensler began a larger activist initiative called "V-Day," focused on eradicating violence against women, bankrolled by the sizeable profits from performances of *The Vagina Monologues*. Without explicit mention of FGCS, V-Day activities have promoted positive body and genital imagery and language, and challenged female genital mutilation (FGM, sometimes called female genital cutting [FGC]).

Petals Project

Nick Karras is a sex educator and photographer who created a video (2005) and a book (2012) of diverse vulva portraits called *The Petals Project* [9]. The anti-FGCS component is made explicit by a quote he places prominently on his website:

Why didn't people tell me about this before I had my labia plasti? I used to really hate the appearance of my inner lips. I was delighted when I originally heard about the labia plasti, so I jumped on it. Yes, they are smaller now and I was pretty happy about it. When I saw this book at my friend's house, I was astonished. This might sound ridiculous, but I really never knew how almost everyone had somewhat large inner lips. After looking at the pictures, I now feel like a circumcised male … it was beautiful as is. It's too late for me, but I hope this book gets to the hands of women around the world who think that having a full labia is not pretty!

Stacy, California. (*all spelling as in original*)

A similar film called *The Centrefold Project* has been showing internationally at women's film festivals and I would guess there are many other similar projects of photography and affirmation. If Jamie McCartney is right, making these films affects participants as well as viewers, destigmatising and demystifying their own "lady bits."

The Muffia

The Muffia is a UK performance art collective of Katie O'Brien and Sinead King, who began making political statements about women's bodies on the streets of London and Manchester in 2008 [10]. They wore furry/hairy pubic muffs (pubic hair wigs known as "merkins") outside their clothes as they walked around, using their bodies as billboards to deliver body liberation messages. While not explicitly about labia or cosmetic surgery, their demonstrations draw attention to being proud "down there," and thus count as a form of FGCS activism.

Visible Vagina Show

An exhibition of vulva art pieces by dozens of prominent artists was shown in 2010 at a New York art gallery [11]. A beautiful catalog was published. Reviews were positive, although generally concurring that the "shock value" of this kind of display would have been greater thirty years earlier. Such art shows (and there are others) presumably increase women's positive feelings toward vulva diversity and their own genitalia, albeit without ever mentioning FGCS.

Activism That Increases FGCS Negatives

Women complained to the UK Advertising Standards Authority about an ad for labiaplasty in the *Metro* newspaper, calling it "irresponsible" and objecting that the description of labiaplasty as achieving "a more natural appearance" implied that presurgery labia might be thought "unnatural" in appearance [12].

Australian investigative television exposed how pornography magazines utilize graphic artists to trim depictions of women's labia to conform to no-genital-details censorship publishing rules. The *Hungry Beast* produced an astonishing video in 2010 showing the similarity of what the graphic artists do to what surgeons do in FGCS, thereby in both cases reducing the types of vulvas to one standard tiny style [13]. Exposing this kind of media trickery presumably increases a negative opinion of FGCS by associating it with deceptive practices.

I will leave it to others in this book to document the gradual increase in restrictive FGCS guidelines developed by various medical groups, only noting that our activism (see later) always included sending letters to such organizations. Though we never received any acknowledgment, it is plausible that our voice helped shift professional judgments.

The FGCS Activism of The New View Campaign

The New View Campaign originated in 2000 to challenge the medicalization of sexuality seen in new dysfunction diagnoses, new biomedical workups for sexual distress, new dysfunction drugs, and the overall incursion of pharmaceutical industry money and medical practitioners into sex research and therapies [14]. We engaged in scholarship such as conferences and publications and activism such as online petitions, op-eds, and public testimony at the U.S. Food and Drug Administration (FDA).

In 2008, we learned of a development in gynecology that seemed tailor-made for our analysis and activism: FGCS. Like the movement of ambitious urologists looking to make a name for themselves in a newly created field of "Female Sexual Dysfunction," a self-identified group of "cosmetogynecologists" was emerging to advertise various FGCS surgical procedures to beautify and "normalize" the vulva. The idea struck us as dangerous to women and designed to exploit women's sexual insecurities and lack of anatomical information. FGCS seemed uncannily similar to the pharmaceutical industry's promoting drugs as the best way to help women's sexual response problems.

Our FGCS activism took place over a four-year period, 2008–2011, involving many different activities and a changing cadre of activists, and as with most amateur activism it evolved as opportunities arose and our analysis expanded.

2008

Our involvement with FGCS began as a result of a 2008 *New York Times* article about a new "pelvic fitness" clinic that referred to "cosmetogynecology" [15,16]. Our small New York City antimedicalization study group decided to research this new industry and to plan some sort of activism. We didn't have a plan of action but our experience with the pharmaceutical industry gave us some directions. The work was done by a core group of five (primarily NYC graduate students in critical psychology) and about a dozen additional helpers and demonstration participants drawn from my feminist friends and colleagues. All of our actions and research are shown on an extensive webpage we created [17].

We identified eight New York City cosmetogynecologists who advertised FGCS procedures online and made a chart of information from their websites (e.g., the types of procedures on offer, whether they were franchisees of entrepreneurial California surgeon David Matlock who promoted FGCS as a business, if they showed before-and-after photos, etc.). We documented the "exaggerated and misleading claims" made on the websites. We wrote ten letters to US government officials and agencies (e.g., Federal Trade Commission Office of Consumer Affairs [FTC]) and professional organizations (e.g., American College of Obstetrics and Gynecology [ACOG]) protesting the unregulated advertising and claimsmaking we observed. We did not receive a single reply.

Pretending to be prospective patients, we visited the clinics and chose one with a location that seemed appropriate for a street demonstration. We sent a press release to hundreds of media outlets announcing our action to demand attention to the effects of unregulated surgical procedures on women's labia and vaginas. We obtained more than fifty endorsers of our demonstration and posted their names online. We scheduled an afternoon of sign-making at The New School University and prepared costumes for our guerrilla theater piece. We notified the police of our planned demonstration and they set up sawhorses to confine our march to a limited part of the sidewalk.

Our two-hour street demonstration in November (chilly but sunny) consisted in walking in a circle on the sidewalk outside the office building housing Dr. Ronald Blatt's FGCS office chanting slogans and carrying colorful signs reading, for example, "Long Live Long Labia," "Stop Marketing Discontent" and "More Research Less Marketing" (see Figures 10.1 and 10.2). Three members of our group repeatedly performed a guerrilla theater piece titled "Dr. IFFA and the Two

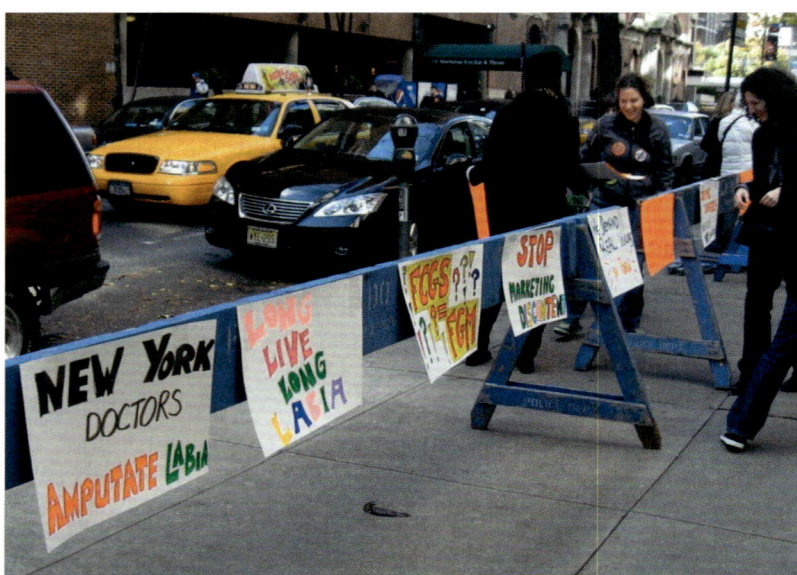

Figure 10.1 New View campaign.

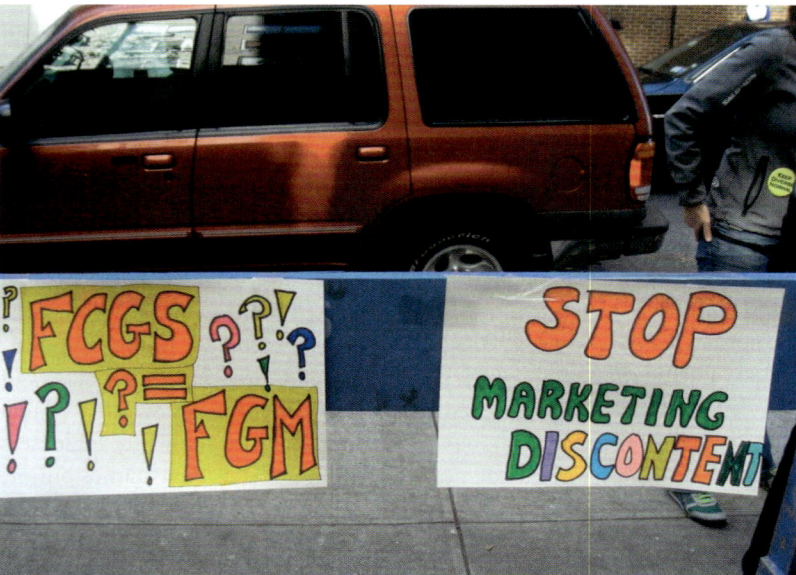

Figure 10.2 FCGS street demonstration in New York City, November 2008.

Labias" highlighting the seductive interest-free financing (IFFA) policies of cosmetogynecology doctors. We compiled still photos into a one-minute video. Our demonstration was covered in *TIME* magazine [18] as well as being written up by demonstration members in various publications and blogs.

2009

Following our street demonstration, which we filed under "increasing the negatives" of FGCS, we decided to turn to "decreasing the positives" and learn about the pro-vulva movement and the uses of art in activism. We elected to have a weekend gallery exhibit and looked for a long time for an appropriate venue (an empty storefront, for example, or a university gallery). We finally found an affordable space in Brooklyn, "The Change You Want To See Gallery," that was used for casual co-working during the week and could be rented for a weekend [19]. We contacted local artists who could easily bring their vulva art to Brooklyn (photos, paintings, videos, knitted and crocheted vulvas, books, puppets, etc.). All the artists are listed on the project webpage along with a final report [20]. After setting up all day Saturday, the event began with a Saturday night wine, cheese, and dj music party.

Our event poster displayed vulva drawings originally made by artist-turned-sexuality-educator Betty Dodson. In addition to the vulva-positive art on the gallery walls and tables, we photocopied vulva outlines from Dodson's pioneering pro-masturbation books [21,22] and provided crayons for people to color them in. On the reverse side of each vulva drawing was a letter inviting college and university women's and gender studies programs to help organize local events to further celebrate women's genital diversity. Each person who colored in a vulva gave us the name of a college program, and we mailed out several dozen of the drawings/letters. We did not receive a single reply to these mailings.

Through word of mouth and descriptive flyers left at many coffee shops and bookstores, we had a large turnout and speedily went through three cases of wine. We stopped during the party briefly to honor Betty Dodson for her many contributions to women's sexual emancipation, and linked the gallery event to our larger campaign against medicalization and FGCS.

We reconfigured the gallery on Sunday with a seminar table in the middle of the room for a "brunch salon" with bagels and speakers. The theme was resistance to accurate depiction of genital diversity and how it lays the groundwork for FGCS. The walls were still hung with vulva artworks. Jon Knowles, Director of Public Education at Planned Parenthood, discussed his organization's ambivalence to explicit genital imagery in their literature. Svetlana Mintcheva from the National Coalition Against Censorship discussed nationwide restrictions around nudity and genital imagery in public spaces. New View Campaign member Meika Loe facilitated the discussion among walk-in attendees as well as a busload of her women's studies students from Colgate University in upstate New York. Again we had a huge crowd all day taking selfies in front of the artworks and coloring in vulvas until we closed the gallery in the late afternoon.

The total expenses for the event (rental, food, printing, hanging materials, etc.) came to about $1900. A five-minute video that shows the event including the art, poster and opening night party is on YouTube [23]. Although we received no replies from our college letters, the attendees were very enthusiastic about the exhibition, and filled our guest book with positive comments. I often wonder how widely all those selfies were distributed. The initial shock that people reflected (in giggles) on entering the gallery subsided rapidly until taking selfies seemed fun and unproblematic.

2010

We continued monitoring the cosmetogynecology industry, and when we learned that they were planning an international professional conference in Las Vegas, we planned a "counter-conference" on the campus of the University of Nevada – Las Vegas (UNLV) for the same weekend. This would be the third conference of the New View Campaign and the only one of six wholly about FGCS. The illustrated report of that event is on our New View website [24], as are several of the plenary lectures [25]. Virginia Braun, a New Zealand gender studies professor who had published several analyses of FGCS, was invited to speak at both conferences. Although the FGCS industry was not planning to embrace the insights of social science, nor was it interested in knowing about our "counter-conference" happening uptown, it liked the appearance of multidisciplinarity on its program, and Ginny was able to share with us much up-to-date material she learned about the industry.

Our conference, titled "Framing the Vulva," was planned over a very short ten-week period with the help of colleagues in Women's Studies at UNLV. It lacked advanced registration or any budget for speakers or travel, but we were learning that we could raise awareness and tell stories online as well as through publications or in person. Our type of amateur activism has the advantage of being flexible. About eighty-five people attended, coming from across the United States and Canada. We designed an activist exhibit called "Talk Back to Surgeons" consisting of five large posters on easels with photos and quotes from FGCS surgeons' websites. The easels held note cards, and conference attendees were encouraged to write messages that would be mailed to the surgeons. The project was put online following the conference to recruit additional participants [26].

A full afternoon of workshops allowed the attendees to learn and share activist strategies involving subjects from vulva art to feminist research. In the evening there were exhibits set up in the large Las Vegas Erotic Heritage Museum during a couple of hours of socializing ending with a raffle of sex toys to support the conference. Overall, the conference made it clear to the public and the cosmetogynecologists that their new industry is under widespread surveillance and that critical analyses are emerging from scholar-activists in several disciplines. The direct contact with the industry afforded by Ginny Braun's presentations and the easel talkback project gave participants a sense that the New View Campaign was effective and up-to-date in its activism.

2011

Our fourth and final year of FGCS activism was called "Vulvanomics" and consisted of online projects [27]. Our small New View Campaign team was occupied writing articles for professional journals and planning other antimedicalization conferences, so online activism was a necessity. We started with an online petition calling for more FGCS regulation directed to the FTC and ACOG (as were our letters in 2008), which continues to gather signatures (as of October 2017, more than 1,100) [28].

We created a project called "Flash Activism," whereby on a certain date groups and individuals would take selfie photos holding up protest signs in front of cosmetic genital surgeons' offices. We would make a collage of the resulting photos and upload it to social media [29]. A college group from Ontario in Canada even received local press coverage for their protest. As in previous years, we posted on the event webpage a resource list of up-to date FGCS statistics, recent journalism, and new books that showed the wide range of female genitalia in a celebratory and artistic manner.

The pièce de resistance for 2011 and, in my opinion, our entire FCGS activism was a ten-minute satirical video called "Dr. Vajayjay's! Privatize Those Privates!" that was written, cast, and filmed by our small New York team (and friends) [30]. The bill for this video, including video and editing equipment and room rental, props, food, but no payment to actors (thank you, Michael DeNola, our "dr" star), was about $2,000. Rachel Liebert, CUNY graduate student at the

time and mastermind of "Dr. VJJ," also prepared a study guide that is on the YouTube page. We poured our years of research and analysis about FGCS into "Dr. VJJ," along with all our anger at unscrupulous surgeons, their manipulation of facts, and their masterful promotional strategies. The video is amusing, but also deeply informed.

Satire is a powerful tool for activism, and "Dr. VJJ" is not the only satirical effort to challenge FGCS. The feminist website "Jezebel" offered a sarcastic analysis in 2015 with their advice to get a labiaplasty so you can fit into yoga pants. However, I am sorry to say that the very day I am writing this, the British news had yet another article about the yoga pants "problem" [31]. Australian singer-songwriter Melissa Main posted a hilarious song, "I'm saving up for a designer vagina" on YouTube [32]. YouTube also has some guerrilla female genital cosmetic surgery theater from 2008 called "Welcome to the Designer Vagina Clinic!" [33]. Dr. Dicko and his scissors look just like our Dr. IFFA (Interest Free Financing Available) from our street protest of 2008! Humor is spirit-building, but with "Dr. VJJ" we also attempted to include our analysis of the strategies used by the cosmetogynecology industry.

Conclusion

It is not easy combining academic scholarship and activism into one career [34]. Activism takes much time and effort and I have given considerable detail in this chapter to convey some of that. Academic reward structures do not acknowledge or reward activism in terms of recognition, promotion, or tenure. As activism is unpaid work, it has to compete with paid speeches and book royalties, as well as paid employment. The primary incentives for activism come from living one's values, along with the pleasures of political collaboration and engaging in self-directed activities. For me, as well, there have been the rewards of intergenerational teamwork and intellectual discussion.

The primary problem, however, is not missing out on conventional academic rewards; it's that activist training for academics is largely on-the-job learning and self-taught scholar-activists such as myself constantly feel inadequate. Activists are hungry for insight into the practices and experiences of "real" organizers, into how collective and personal commitment can be sustained, into relationships between day–to-day activism and "long-range vision," etc. Where do we learn this?

References

1. Several pages on http://newviewcampaign.org detail our FGCS work, especially http://newviewcampaign.org/, fgcs.asp, http://newviewcampaign.org/vulvagraphics.asp, http://newviewcampaign.org/conference3.asp, and http://newviewcampaign.org/vulvanomics.asp

2. Croteau D, Hoynes W, Ryan C. Introduction: Integrating social movement theory and practice. In Croteau D, Hoynes W, Ryan C, (eds), *Rhyming hope and history: Activists, academics and social movement scholarship*. Minneapolis: University of Minnesota Press; 2005, pp. xi–xviii.

3. Westermann LB, Oakley SH, Mazloomdoost D, et al. Attitudes regarding labial hypertrophy and labiaplasty: A survey of members of the Society of Gynecologic Surgeons and the North American Society for Pediatric and Adolescent Gynecology. *Female Pelvic Med Reconstr Surg*. 2016;22(3):175–9.

4. Horton K. Stats show labiaplasty is becoming more popular. Available from: www.plasticsurgery.org/news/blog/stats-show-labiaplasty-is-becoming-more-popular

5. Morgan-Davies M. This woman has been holding workshops to design patchwork vaginas out of fabric, fur and glitter. Available from: www.walesonline.co.uk/news/wales-news/woman-been-holding-workshops-design-11009241

6. McCartney J. Great Wall of Vagina. Fine Art Studios. Available from: www.greatwallofvagina.co.uk/home

7. McCartney J. Great Wall of Vagina. Opportunities. Fine Art Studios. Available from: www.greatwallofvagina.co.uk/opportunities

8. *The Vagina Monologues*. Available from: https://en.wikipedia.org/wiki/The_Vagina_Monologues

9. *Petals*. Available from: www.nickkarras.com/petals.html

10. The Muffia. Available from: https://themuffiablog.wordpress.com/

11. The Visible Vagina. David Nolan New York. Available from: www.davidnolangallery.com/exhibitions/the-visible-vagina

12. Advert for London 'designer vagina' surgery banned. Available from: www.bbc.com/news/uk-england-london-36262199

13. Russell A. Labiaplasty. *Hungry Beast*, ABC1. Available from: https://vimeo.com/10883108

14. Tiefer L. Arriving at a "new view" of women's sexual problems: Background, theory, and activism. In Kaschak L, Tiefer L, (eds), *A New View of Women's Sexual Problems*. Binghamton, NY: Haworth; 2001, pp. 63–98;

15. Tiefer L. Still resisting after all these years: An update on sexuo-medicalization and on the New View Campaign to challenge the medicalization of women's sexuality. *Sex Relat Ther*. 2001; 25:189–96.

16. www.nytimes.com/ 192008/07/03/fashion/03SkinOne.html

17. New View Campaign. Available from: www.newviewcampaign.org/fgcs.asp

18. Plastic surgery below the belt. Available from: http://content.time.com/time/health/article/0,8599,1859937,00.html

19. I might point out that 2009 was before Brooklyn was gentrified into a hugely popular destination. At the time of our event, the neighborhood we chose was, shall we say, fairly down and out and hence the venue was affordable.

20. Vulvagraphics: An intervention in honor of female genital diversity. Available from: http://newviewcampaign.org/vulvagraphics.asp

21. Dodson B. *Liberating masturbation*. New York: Three Rivers Press; 1974.

22. Dodson B. *Sex for one: The joy of selfloving*. New York: Three Rivers Press; 1987.

23. Liebert RJ. Vulvagraphics. Available from: www.youtube.com/watch?v=wuJ37hrWFKI&version=3&hl=en%5FUS&rel=0

24. Framing the vulva: Genital cosmetic surgery and genital diversity. Available from: www.newviewcampaign.org/userfiles/file/Final%20Report%20revised.pdf

25. New View's videos. Available from: https://vimeo.com/user5043385/videos

26. Talking back to the maketing of women's sexualities. https://newviewcampaignblog.wordpress.com/

27. Vulvanomics. Available from: www.newviewcampaign.org/vulvanomics.asp

28. Pleasure not profits! Available from: https://petitions.moveon.org/sign/pleasure-not-profits

29. www.newviewcampaign.org/media/pdfs/Flash%20Activism.pdf

30. Dr. Vajayjay's! Privatize those privates! www.youtube.com/watch?v=T9kCw0Lmaa0

31. No more camel (toe) pose! www.dailymail.co.uk/fema il/article-4971584/Women-seek-vaginal-surgery-look-better-yoga-pants.html

32. Designer vagina song by Melissa Main. www.youtube .com/watch?v=dHQ_mMFpDsI

33. The designer vagina clinic. www.youtube.com/watch? v=HJPLHeF_SDw

34. Cancian FM. Conflicts between activist research and academic success: Participatory research and alternative strategies. *Am Sociol.* 1993;24:92–106.

Can Better Sex Education Tackle the Rise in Female Genital Cosmetic Surgery?

Tove Lundberg

Can "comprehensive sex education" [1, p. 475] tackle the dissatisfaction and distress that underpin female genital cosmetic surgery (FGCS)? A literature search has not identified any research that can directly answer the question, nor has it turned up resources that sex educators can immediately put to use. Nevertheless, theories developed within sex education (sex ed) can have useful applications for addressing female genital concerns and FGCS.

My understanding of sex ed is framed by my position as a norm-critical clinical psychologist with a specialist focus in sexology. A Swedish-speaking Finlander, I completed my clinical psychology training in Sweden and doctoral research training in Norway and now live and work in Sweden near the border with Denmark. I draw on my understanding of sex ed in Sweden to explore the topic in question.

Despite a relatively liberal attitude to sex ed in Sweden, several reports have concluded that provision is patchy and that the quality is inconsistent between schools and between teachers [2]. Many programmes aim at fostering well-being and equal (sexual) relationships but end up mainly giving information on fertility and sexually transmitted infections (STIs) [3]. Further development is undoubtedly required in Sweden and the rest of Scandinavia to meet new and emergent challenges, such as the issues that steer women towards FGCS. Nevertheless, useful lessons can be drawn from the Swedish sex ed context.

The chapter begins with a brief introduction to sex ed and discusses how programmes could be expanded to become more *comprehensive*. The discussion progresses to more specific deliberations to situate pedagogic responses to female genital distress within a feminist and norm-critical framework. Whereas women are steered by normative pressures to ask what they can do for their genitals, effective norm-critical sex ed could help more women to reverse the question by asking what their genitals can do for them.

A Brief Introduction of Sex Education

Sex ed is mandatory in many post-industrial nations where school attendance is compulsory for children. That said, it is contested in most countries, if not conflicted to the point of stagnation. Suffice to say that there are strong ideological drivers behind the questions as to whether sex ed does more harm than good, what the content should be, how should it be taught, who should teach it, and how old the children or adolescents should be when they participate in it. The prevailing ideas, influenced by strong social values, can be thought of as falling into conservative, liberal and feminist/postmodern perspectives [4]. Conservative approaches typically focus on fostering abstinence from sexual activities before marriage. Liberal approaches are oriented towards promoting a shame-free attitude to sex and sexuality and emphasizing sexual rights and sexual health. Feminist critics, however, argue that in reality, such liberal approaches usually fail to foster positive and agentic sexualities [3]. In practice, most sex ed programmes probably reflect shades of grey in between these three broad orientations.

Traditional sex ed programmes use didactic methods to teach young people to evade the negative consequences of sexual activities such as pregnancies and/or STIs. Critics suggest that such a negative focus fails to engage young people as sexual agents [3] and homogenises them [4]. Such limitations have particular ramifications for young women and gender and sexual minorities. For example, the conflation of sex and coitus and reproduction is based on cis- and hetero-normative assumptions and leaves little room for other possibilities. Advocates argue that feminist and LGBTQI perspectives should not be applied to mainstream sex ed as *add-ons* but transform it altogether by addressing complex psychosocial aspects of bodies, identities, relationships, desires and norms.

Evidence-based sex ed programmes require the collaborative involvement of interdisciplinary stakeholders to develop clear aims and content [5–7]. Research also suggests that programmes should include theoretical information about social influence, delivered in group-based methods informed by cognitive and developmental theories. Such group exercises can enable participants to reflect on what the information might mean to them personally but also to access each other's perspectives. Young people also have opportunities to reflect on how best to counter the effect of unhelpful social influences and acquire social interaction skills to navigate sexual situations. As such the processing of information and its translation in lived realities might qualify such sex ed approaches as *comprehensive*. Although the programmes that have been evaluated have targeted specific behaviours, such as preventing transmission of HIV/AIDS, the insights gained from delivery of these programmes are relevant for distressed and dissatisfied girls and women seeking FGCS.

In Sweden, sex ed has been a mandatory part of the school curriculum since 1955 [8]. The guidelines issued by the Swedish National Agency for Education recommend that sex ed is introduced from age 6 and an integrated part of most subjects [4]. From age 6 to 9, for example, biology lessons should focus on not just how the body appears and functions but also the importance of relationships on overall well-being. From age 10 and onwards, questions concerning puberty, sexuality, reproduction, identity, relationships, love, equality and responsibility should be introduced and integrated in a range of subjects [9]. In addition to integrating sex ed in all subjects, teachers are encouraged to have specific hours devoted to sex ed and address questions related to sexuality whenever they are raised in class – regardless of subject. Having moved from social non-inclusiveness to a tolerance-based perspective on LGBT sexualities, Swedish sex ed is, according to some authors, embracing a norm-critical approach as articulated in the guidelines provided by the Swedish National Agency for Education [4]. Despite these guidelines, however, reports suggest that the principles do not always translate consistently into practice [2].

Although sex ed is typically delivered to pupils in schools as part of a broader public health agenda, aspects of sex ed can be adapted to other settings [5, 10]. Health care providers, for example, can usefully deploy aspects of socially inclusive sex ed to meet patient needs in various clinical specialties. For example, sexual difficulties are associated with progressed diabetes; therefore a discussion of non-coital/penetrative sexual activities can be a useful aspect of diabetes care and counselling delivered by nurse specialists (see Chapter 14, this volume). However, research shows that health care providers are in general poorly trained to talk about sex and sexuality with patients in a helpful and confident manner [11]. Building on these insights, the World Health Organization etc. The World Health Organization (WHO) argues that sex ed should be integrated into the professional education of health care providers [10].

Despite conceptual shifts in sex ed to focus more on well-being rather than risks and diseases, many sex ed programmes are still focused on providing information that focus on the latter [10]. Workers continue to argue for information to become much more comprehensive to help young people to make choices about their bodies and lives in the social sphere [2]. Several commentators have also suggested that such comprehensive provision of information would constitute an important response to the problems that underpin the seeking of FGCS [12]. In the text that follows, I outline how sex ed could include information to address the rising problem of FGCS but also discuss the limits of information giving, however well put together.

Information on Female Genital Appearance Diversity

In traditional sex ed materials, the female genitalia are usually discussed within a narrative of threat. The vagina, represented as a desensitised, inanimate recess, is typically emphasised over and above the rest of the genital anatomy [3]. Images are usually clinical and factual, often with an internal rather than an external view. If the external genitalia are represented at all they are seldom erect and present. Outside sex ed, in some mass media and mainstream pornography, the female genital anatomy is portrayed as a flat and smooth surface with a vertical slit that gives the two sides perfect symmetry [13]. Within medicine, there is a lack of descriptions of genital appearance diversity [14]. In the context of increased exposure of the female genitalia via modern genital grooming techniques and revealing clothing, many girls and women not surprisingly find themselves feeling anxious and confused as to how their genitals (should) look (to others). In a social context where female body image distress is already rife and where intense marketing of unproven medical interventions is permitted, if not encouraged, it is unsurprising that many girls and women judge themselves against the homogenised aesthetic being sold [15, 16].

In health and social care, where dilemmatic issues appear, people typically call for more information. However, information on the diversity of female genital appearance and structure to counter the above is not exactly lacking. Rather, materials are not utilized or even subjugated. Since the 1970s, feminists have encouraged women to do self-examinations in order to get to know and appreciate their vulvas [17]. Newer resources such as the Labia Library and The Great Wall of Vagina are easily accessible to enhance sex ed programmes. However, some information and materials are easily absorbed while others have very little currency, depending on the prevailing narratives and norms, and it is the unhelpful narratives and norms that should be the focus of interventions [18].

Pedagogic theorists have been at stake at emphasising the limits of instructing people via information alone [19]. Many sex educators and health professionals have experienced the limits of *teaching as instruction* that ignores the contextually dependent and interactional aspects of learning [20]. Early on, pedagogic experts have pointed out that learning is a matter not of instruction but construction [21]. Factual information targets cognitions, not emotions. In an interview study, the authors highlighted that several of their participants reported that they *knew* that female genitals came in a variety of shapes and sizes but that such knowledge did not affect the negative *feelings* that they had about their genitalia [16]. Telling girls and women about diversity may modify their knowledge but usually fails to shift the negative, albeit false and socially constructed, meaning of genital protrusion in females. It is the meaning that distresses the individuals [13]. Psychosocial interventions can be useful precisely because they centralise emotions and work to transform meaning [22]. Overall, it is the social construction of the female genital anatomy as an invisible recess (hence it is typically called a vagina) that needs to be challenged collectively. Finally, focusing on information on appearance diversity could even reify the importance of genital appearance. As long as appearance *matters*, feelings, including shame and pride, will be highly invested in it (see Chapter 3 by Braun, this volume).

It has been suggested that interventions could promote 'vulvar literacy' [27, p. 145] among women.

Research suggests that genital dissatisfaction is a driver in FGCS [16, 23] and that this is not easily accounted for. For example, mainstream pornography is associated with an openness to labiaplasty, but the relationship is not usually a linear one [24]. Studies show that women seeking labiaplasty have internalised representations of the genitalia from the internet and advertisements [23]. Watching images of modified vulvas seems to affect what general young women perceive as normal and desirable [25]. If women's internal representations of normal and desirable vulvas are modifiable by watching media images, might not these representations shift via counter-exposures [15, 26]?

The Swedish Association for Sexuality Education (RFSU) encourages sex educators to draw external and erect genitals and allow different genitals to be represented in drawings, for example, genitals of different sizes that may be symmetrical and less symmetrical and sometimes with and sometimes without hair. Furthermore, norm-critical pedagogical exercises are recommended whereby participants are asked to articulate all kinds of "genital language" that they know [8]. Participants are then asked to critically discuss the connotations of different words as well as the limitations and possibilities of each term. They are also encouraged to explore language that could be useful in different contexts in order to develop a bank of possible terms to use in sexual and non-sexual situations. In relation to FGCS, some commentators have suggested that health professionals also need to develop different ways of talking about genitals. One important issue is to develop language that avoids making sense of appearance in dichotomies (e.g., normal versus abnormal, small versus large) [28].

In summary, although information on genital diversity is an important response to the distress that underpins FGCS, insights from sex ed also point to the risks of becoming over-invested in informational resources. These concerns are supportive of two conceptual shifts already occurring in sex ed in some quarters. First of all, the focus is being redirected from needs to rights and from disease to pleasure [10]. Second, the ideological underpinning of sex ed is increasingly debated. Commentators argue, for example, that a focus on information often implies a neoliberal understanding of individual agency [28], and some raise the question if this is the *kind of agent* that sex educators should foster. Critical scholars suggest that we move from a focus on information to an exploration of the kinds of agency we should promote [3].

Promoting Personal Agency

Refocusing from information to agency does not mean discarding the works discussed earlier. Rather, we need to interrogate the ideological and theoretical underpinnings of sex ed and evaluate the consequences of sex ed programmes. For example, on reviewing a sex ed programme, we can ask: what opportunities for personal agency does this programme open up and close down? This kind of critical engagement with personal agency has been demonstrated in sex ed [3] and in interventions that specifically target the problem of FGCS [28]. In this section, I explore alternative ways of thinking about agency in sex ed but also discuss the limitations of focusing on agency.

Exposing the Gendered Misappropriation of Agency

Feminist scholars argue that the intention to provide young people with information to make choices is grounded in a liberal ideology but reflects a simplistic understanding of individuals as rational agents and negates the importance of social structures and power relations. Such an understanding of choice is stripped of our gendered social context (see Chapter 8 by Chambers, this volume). It is problematic to talk about an autonomous individual freely choosing a potentially harmful intervention in a context where social and media pressure to live up to certain ideals is inescapable and experienced daily [28]. Critical commentators suggest that we focus on the available discursive resources within our social, cultural and economic contexts within which 'choice' is freely made.

How then, could sex ed help to promote *agency* that would enable people to become sexual and embodied agents in *new* ways? In feminist and critical education, such agency is fostered not by information on what people *do* and *are*, but by exploring what people *can do* and *can become* [3]. This move from a descriptive to a *transformative* stance is similar to the goals of norm-critical approaches. Norm-critical sex ed examines "different societal norms and how they affect people on an individual, group and societal level. The aim is to notice and challenge the norms that frame what is considered 'normal' and thus what is, unconsciously, understood as desirable" [29, p. 23].

Norm-critical sex ed therefore aims at creating spaces of becoming [30], where young people are encouraged to move from questions such as *what they can do for their genitals* to fit with normative understandings of sex and sexuality, to a focus on *what their genitals can do for them*. Some ways of providing such spaces of becoming are explored next.

Sexuality as 'a Central Aspect of Being Human'

Norm-critical workers suggest that we draw on more holistic conceptualisations of sexuality in sex ed that position sexuality as "a central aspect of being human" [31, p. 5]. Sexuality should therefore always be included in all interventions aimed at promoting overall well-being. Sexuality should also be addressed with a broad focus: that talking about sexuality is more than just addressing sexual activities or talking about genitals. Similar to commentators suggesting that feminist and LGBTQI perspectives can help transform sex ed altogether, I suggest that the information to address genital distress should not only be applied as an add-on, but that such distress should bring transformational potential to sex ed. I interpret the genital discomfort that young people experience as a sign that sex ed as a whole is not meeting their needs and requires change.

The understanding that sexuality is a central aspect of being human also makes integration of sex ed in all school subjects reasonable. In Sweden, several guidelines have been developed to assist teachers in the endeavour of making sex ed part of everyday teaching. One example is Sex in School [9], which was developed in an interprofessional collaboration between representatives from education, health care, sex ed and RFSU. This material outlines age-appropriate and specific themes and questions that teachers can consider in relation to each specific school subject. Some examples are presented and discussed next. I will draw on this material as an example and discuss how such ways of working also can be used to address genital discomfort.

In Sweden, subjects such as Citizenship should provide a space to develop *critical thinking*. In Sex in School [9], it is suggested that such critical thinking in Citizenship can be connected to History. For example, students can develop a timeline to outline the historical shifts in sexuality narratives. Students are asked to explore and discuss how historical understandings, legislation and media representations frame how we understand 'normal' sexuality today by examining what counted and still counts as 'normal' sexual behaviour and how freedom of action was and is gendered and dependent on other factors such as age and class.

In the same vein, students are likewise invited to explore how people have, and still are, resisting and negotiating norms. This could entail analysing the strategies that feminists and the LGBTQI or Black Lives Matter movements have used and are utilising in struggles for liberation and human rights. These exercises could further be developed by creating spaces where student-led resistance could be identified and further explored. It might include encouragement to take part in, or organise, subcultures where alternative and empowering norms could appear. More current work in schools could involve analysing social media campaigns such as #meeto in order to understand how individual shame and silence can be transformed socially and collectively to create resistance.

Both RFSU and Sex in School suggest that sex ed related to Biology should include not just fertility but also anatomy and bodily sensitivity and responsiveness [8, 9]. Talking norm-critically about anatomy requires the sex educator to know the problems and limits of mainstream anatomical knowing as well as the history of anatomy (see Chapter 2 by Crouch, this volume). In Sex in School the authors suggest that the norm-critical way of focusing on anatomy involves exploring similarities between male and female genitals rather than their differences and focusing on variations of appearance and functioning beyond the standard message. Biology is seen as a subject that could provide opportunities to talk about different dimensions of sex and gender (such as biological, legal, psychological and social) and different ways of becoming a parent – rather than focusing on mechanistic representations of the body and reproduction.

RFSU typically start their norm-critical sex ed with exercises where participants are asked to discuss *what sex is* [8]. This is another example of how critical thinking skills can be invoked to question taken-for-granted understandings that frame the way we think about ourselves and sexuality. Such exercises aim at creating further discussions about biological, psychological and sociological aspects that are personally relevant to the participants. To target genital concerns or distress, these exercises could be extended to include a more explicit focus on gender and the

body. Such exercises could get participants even more involved in questioning the idealised body and challenge prevailing norms by asking: How do we, and could we, think about our bodies? Do we treat it like a passive surface, a symbol or something else [32]? What consequences do these approaches have on our thinking about our bodies and how we work them? Similarly, we could think critically about our genitals and question the taken-for-granted understanding that the main purpose of genitals is procreation or heterosexual performance, by asking what our genitals can do for us. Such questioning of biology might encourage new ways to think and act in relation to our genitals. Such discussions also connect with classroom exercises whereby students are asked to critically explore how sexual practices, sexual arousal and desire can be understood both as separate and connected [9]. It can also lead to discussions in sex ed of the variations in what makes people feel good and what they desire [33], and how people can respect themselves and others.

Other exercises outlined in Sex in School include using Art and Design to foster critical approaches to media representations, including pornography. Knowledge of Chemistry may stimulate lively debates about what does (sexual) 'chemistry' mean, and how these ideas relate to everyday understandings of what is 'natural' in sex and relationships – for example, is monogamy more 'natural' than polygamy. In Language classes, learners can gain understanding as to how different languages are gendered as well as how young people think about sexuality and sex ed depending on where they live [9]. The aim of all of these exercises is to cultivate a critical understanding of what is normal and desirable and to challenge any prevailing notion as absolute fact. In Sex in School, the authors further suggest that coping with negative feelings could be addressed in Music, for example, how music can be used to cope with bad feelings and accentuate positive feelings [9].

Psychological research suggests that people who experience genital distress may face additional uncertainty in relationships. Thus some researchers have focused upon self-efficacy and self-esteem. However, some commentators suggest that such constructs are problematic [34]. As an alternative, other psychological constructs such as those relating to self-acceptance and self-compassion could be included more explicitly in sex ed. Self-compassion includes cognitive as well as affective aspects and can be understood as acceptance of (instead of judgement against) oneself, feelings of belonging to a common humanity (instead of isolation) and putting feelings in a wider perspective (instead of overidentifying with them). Self-compassion is important in situations in which our efforts are insufficient in a certain situation as well as in general life situations that are difficult to bear. Fostering self-compassion could be an interesting way of responding to oppressive and unrealistic norms as well as coping with shame and fear of rejection.

It can be argued that adolescence is far too late to learn to interrogate the social contexts, especially when the young people are emotionally overwhelmed by body image distress. Several programmes suggest that young children can develop critical philosophical skills [35] and from interventions to prevent the development of body image distress in relation to weight and eating [36]. Judging from such research, the foundations of body image are laid in childhood [37]. Girls are also pressured to live up to an adult body ideal earlier than boys. In other words, interventions that focus on factors such as body image and bodily integrity [38] need to start long before puberty.

The Problems and Limits of Focusing on Personal Agency

The problem of FGCS cannot be resolved by a focus on the individual. Parallel steps have to be taken to tackle the social structure that frames individual choices [28]. Some feminist scholars argue that *agency* works on the assumption that individuals are (to a greater or lesser extent) rational and critical. This remains an assumption and is a problem. Some theorists use feminist and queer understandings of affect to overcome the dualism between the individual and the structure [39]. In combination with perspectives that understand the body as more than just a symbolic surface to improve and make-over [32], interventions may need to work to reconfigure the relationship between individual and social structure.

Is Comprehensive Sex Education Possible?

I have argued that another way of addressing the psychosocial distress underpinning FGCS would be to foster critical thinking by providing opportunities to challenge the taken-for-granted understandings of body and sexuality. Again, there are myriad resources that could assist sex educators to (continue to) do this work. While a focus on agency holds some promise, it may not overcome the challenges that the rising number of FGCS procedures reflect about our social structures. There are a number of reasons for this supposition. First of all, it is important to acknowledge that interventions that target critical agency are at their infancy and will continue to require significant theoretical and practical development, which in turn is based on our collective commitment. It is not clear to what extent any nation is collectively ready for the level of commitment required. A common response from professionals to the idea of norm-critical approaches is 'yet another thing to have to do,' even though it is more about doing the same thing differently. At least in Sweden, there is no lack of articulation on what norm-critical sex ed might look like. The problem lies in putting theory into practice.

To promote sexual health and wellbeing, including genital satisfaction or acceptance, work needs to be done in several domains simultaneously. It is valuable to equip the citizens of tomorrow in sex ed with critical skills and nurture their readiness to resist and negotiate problematic norms. However, approaches to challenge delimiting normativity are also required. The WHO acknowledges that complementary systemic actions across domains such as education as well as law, social policy and health care economics are key in promoting sexual health and well-being in any given community [10]. Systemic measures could include, for example, media codes of conduct [22] and promoting cultural expressions, such as art, literature, films and cartoons, that reframe dominant and limiting discourses (see Chapter 10 by Tiefer, this volume).

Summary

Interventions targeting information such as those on genital appearance diversity are relevant but not sufficient to address the psychosocial drivers of FGCS. They over-rely on simplistic understandings of how information works (or, rather, does not work). Workers who operate within norm-critical understandings of sex ed suggest that education should focus on examining and challenging societal norms with the aim of recognising and disrupting notions of normal and desirable. Norm-critical sex education further encourages a broad focus on body and sexuality by including biological, psychological and sociological aspects in programmes. A focus on biology can include fertility, but should also include aspects such as clitoral anatomy, sensitivity and responsiveness. Psychological aspects should include identity, body image, relationships, communication, and self-compassion. Sociological aspects should cover information about societal norms and social pressure. Norm-critical programmes typically start with exercises where participants are encouraged to challenge commonsense understandings. Such exercises aim at creating further discussions about biological, psychological and sociological aspects that are relevant to participants themselves.

It is as yet unclear if this type of comprehensive sex ed can effectively tackle the cultural, economic and psychological drivers behind FGCS. Drawing on insights highlighted by the WHO, parallel and complementary interventions need to take place in multiple domains, including in legislation, social policies and health and social care infrastructures in order to promote sexual health and well-being including genital satisfaction. Where there is collective action such as that recommended by the WHO, the research and scholarship briefly summarised in this chapter suggest that a norm-critical framework, if allowed to be translated into practice, can provide young people with spaces where they can explore different ways of thinking about their genitals, sexuality and personhood. Rather than focusing on how to make the genitals 'better', 'right', 'acceptable', or 'perfect', more people, from a younger age, may have acquired the skills to flip over to a different type of thinking that focuses on how they can enjoy and appreciate their genitals.

References

1. Tiefer L. Female genital cosmetic surgery: Freakish or inevitable? Analysis from medical marketing, bioethics, and feminist theory. *Fem Psychol.* 2008;18:466–79.

2. Parker R, Wellings K, Lazarus JV. Sexuality education in Europe: An overview of current policies. *Sex Educ.* 2009;9:227–42.

3. Allen L. Beyond the birds and the bees: Constituting a discourse of erotics in sexuality education. *Gend Educ.* 2004;16:151–67.

4. Sherlock L. Sociopolitical influences on sexuality education in Sweden and Ireland. *Sex Educ.* 2012;12:383–96.

5. Kirby D. *No easy answers: Research findings on programs to reduce teen pregnancy.* Washington, DC: National Campaign to Prevent Teen Pregnancy; 1997.

6. Ross DA, Dick B, Ferguson J. Preventing HIV/AIDS in young people: A systematic review of the evidence from developing countries. 2006. Available from: www.unicef.org/aids/files/PREVENTING_HIV_AIDS_IN_YOUNG_PEOPLE__A_SYSTEMATIC_REVIEW_OF_THE_EVIDENCE_FROM_DEVELOPING_COUNTRIES_WHO_2006.pdf

7. Grunseit A, Kippax S. Impact of HIV and sexual health education on the sexual behaviour of young people: A review update. 1997. Available from: www.unaids.org/en/resources/documents/1998/19980421_jc010-impactyoungpeople_en.pdf

8. Skarpås E. Dundermycket sexualundervisning: Falluckor och positiva resultat i ett försök att göra teori till praktik [Loads of sex education: Trapdoors and positive results in an attempt to make theory into practice]. 2010. Available from: www.rfsu.se/Bildbank/Lokalt/Malmo/dokument/Dundermycket_web.pdf?epslanguage=sv

9. Abrahamsson K, Andersson C, Ehinger A, et al. *Sex i skolan [Sex in school].* Ödeshög, Danagårds; 2013.

10. WHO. Developing sexual health programmes: A framework for action. 2010. Available from: http://apps.who.int/iris/bitstream/10665/70501/1/WHO_RHR_HRP_10.22_eng.pdf

11. Dyer K, das Nair R. Why don't healthcare professionals talk about sex? A systematic review of recent qualitative studies conducted in the United Kingdom. *J Sex Med.* 2013;10:2658–70.

12. Cain JM, Iglesia CB, Dickens B, Montgomery O. Body enhancement through female genital cosmetic surgery creates ethical and rights dilemmas. *Int J Gynaecol Obstet.* 2013;122: 169–72.

13. Liao LM, Creighton SM. Requests for cosmetic genitoplasty: How should healthcare providers respond? *BMJ.* 2007;334: 1090.

14. Andrikopoulou M, Michala L, Creighton SM, Liao LM. The normal vulva in medical textbooks. *J Obstet Gynaecol.* 2013;33: 648–50.

15. Laan E, Martoredjo DK, Hesselink S, Snijders N, van Lunsen RH. Young women's genital self-image and effects of exposure to pictures of natural vulvas. *J Psychosom Obstet Gynaecol.* 2016:1–7.

16. Bramwell R, Morland C, Garden AS. Expectations and experience of labial reduction: A qualitative study. *BJOG.* 2007;114: 1493–9.

17. Braun V. The women are doing it for themselves: The rhetoric of choice and agency around female genital cosmetic surgery. *Aust Feminist Stud.* 2009;24:233–49.

18. Foucault M, Gordon C. *Power/knowledge: Selected interviews and other writings, 1972–1977.* New York: Pantheon Books; 1980.

19. Kumashiro KK. Toward a theory of anti-oppressive education. *Rev Educ Res.* 2000;70:25–53.

20. Sullivan Palincsar A. Social constructivist perspectives on teaching and learning. *Annu Rev Psychol.* 1998;49:345–75.

21. Cho S. *Critical pedagogy and social change: Critical analysis on the language of possibility.* New York: Routledge; 2013.

22. The Royal Australian College of General Practitioners. Female genital cosmetic surgery: A resource for general practitioners and other health professionals. 2015. Available from: www.racgp.org.au/download/Docum ents/Guidelines/Female-genital-cosmetic-surgery-tool kit.pdf

23. Sharp G, Tiggemann M, Mattiske J. Factors that influence the decision to undergo labiaplasty: Media, relationships, and psychological well-being. *Aesthet Surg J.* 2016;36:469–78.

24. Jones B, Nurka C. Labiaplasty and pornography: A preliminary investigation. *Porn Studies.* 2015;2:62–75.

25. Moran C, Lee C. What's normal? Influencing women's perceptions of normal genitalia: An experiment involving exposure to modified and nonmodified images. *BJOG.* 2014;121: 761–6.

26. Sharp G, Tiggemann M. Educating women about normal female genital appearance variation. *Body Image.* 2016;16: 70–8.

27. Paarlberg KM, van de Wiel HB. A young woman asking for labia reduction surgery: A plea for 'vulvar literacy'. In Paarlberg KM, van de Wiel HB (eds), *Bio-psycho-social obstetrics and Gynecology: A Competency-Oriented Approach.* Cham, Springer; 2017, pp. 145–63.

28. Braun V. Female genital cosmetic surgery: A critical review of current knowledge and contemporary debates. *J Womens Health.* 2010;19:1393–1407.

29. RFSU. Idéprogram [Conteptual Program]. Stockholm: RFSU [the Swedish Association for Sexuality Education]; 2016.

30. Fields J, Payne E. Editorial introduction: Gender and sexuality taking up space in schooling. *Sex Educ.* 2016;16:1–7.

31. WHO. Defining sexual health: Report of a technical consultation on sexual health, 28–31 January 2002. 2006. Availlable from: www.who.int/reproductive health/publications/sexual_health/defining_sexual_ health.pdf

32. Reischer E, Koo KS. The body beautiful: Symbolism and agency in the social world. *Annu Rev Anthropol.* 2004;33: 297–317.

33. Lamb S, Lustig K, Graling K. The use and misuse of pleasure in sex education curricula. *Sex Educ.* 2013;13:305–18.

34. Neff KD. The role of self-compassion in development: A healthier way to relate to oneself. *Hum Dev.* 2009;52:211–14.

35. Trickey S, Topping KJ. 'Philosophy for children': A systematic review. *Res Papers Educ.* 2004;19: 365–80.

36. Neumark-Sztainer D, Levine MP, Paxton SJ, Smolak L, Piran N, Wertheim EH. Prevention of body dissatisfaction and disordered eating: What next? *Eat Disord.* 2006;14:265–85.

37. Smolak L. Body image in children and adolescents: Where do we go from here? *Body Image.* 2004;1: 15–28.

38. RFSU. *Barns Sexualitet – En Vägledning [Children's sexuality – A guide].* Stockholm: RFSU [the Swedish Association for Sexuality Education], 2015.

39. Ahmed S. *The cultural politics of emotion.* Edinburgh: Edinburgh University Press; 2014.

Female Genital Cosmetic Surgery and the Role of the General Practitioner

Magdalena Simonis

Introduction

The surge in requests for female genital cosmetic surgery (FGCS) has occurred in the context of broader sociocultural developments that encourage the objectification of women's bodies. Of all cosmetic surgeries performed, around 90% are on healthy women who seek surgery to match their aesthetic ideals and elevate their self-esteem. In light of this, the need for health professionals to manage requests for FGCS from a biopsychosocial perspective, with women of all ages, is increasingly present [1].

A confident and knowledgeable general practitioner (GP) who has an understanding of the range of human diversity, but also knows the range of FGCS procedures and their associated risks, is well placed to reassure a patient by first letting her know that, like that of our other physical features, 'normal' genital anatomy varies widely, and can provide education while exploring the deeper issues that may underlie such a request. The GP, the obstetrician/gynaecologist, the plastic and reconstructive surgeon, the urologist and the cosmetic surgeon may differ in the way such requests are dealt with; however, as with all other medical presentations, the medical axiom 'First do no harm' should guide the health professional [2].

What Is FGCS?

The Range of FGCS

The umbrella term FGCS, also known as 'vulvoplasty', encompasses a range of cosmetic procedures aimed at surgically modifying the external and/or internal female genitalia for non-medical reasons, which may be either functional or aesthetic [3]. The most common request is for labiaplasty, which involves the trimming of the inner lips or labia minora. Labiaplasty may be combined with trimming or removal of the clitoral hood to expose the clitoris and to create even labia minora that do not protrude

beyond the line of the outer lips – the labia majora. The desirability of this genital appearance has increased among women partly as a result of sociocultural changes such as the accessibility of online images that have been airbrushed, online pornography, changes in fashion and the increasing trend for genital hair removal which exposes anatomy with which women and girls are unfamiliar [4].

The terms labiaplasty, vulvoplasty and FGCS are often used interchangeably, although most requests are for labiaplasty. Vulvoplasty can include labiaplasty, clitoral hood reduction or removal, mons pubis fat injections or liposuction. Hymenoplasty, colloquially referred to as 'revirgination', is sought by women of certain cultural backgrounds where virginity is valued or in existing relationships as a 'gift' to one's partner. 'G-shot' involves autologous fat or collagen transfer via injection into a pre-determined 'G-spot' location. There is no existing scientific literature describing this procedure. 'Orgasm-shot' is described as a sexual and cosmetic rejuvenation procedure for the vagina using the preparation and injection of blood-derived growth factors into the G-spot, clitoris and labia [5]. 'Vaginal rejuvenation' can either be delivered through the use of a fractionated CO_2 laser, or surgically. Perineoplasty, which involves the reinforcement of the pelvic floor sometimes performed with vaginal tightening, or vaginoplasty, is also referred to as 'surgical vaginal rejuvenation'. This has been performed for post-birth stress urinary incontinence (SUI) or pelvic organ prolapse (POP). Traditionally, however, in this context it is performed to allegedly enhance sexual pleasure for both partners by increasing friction with penile thrust during coitus.

Incidence of FGCS

The first labiaplasty procedure reported was in 1987 in the USA, and by 2014 labiaplasty was listed in the

USA as the fourth most common aesthetic surgical procedure following liposuction, rhinoplasty and breast augmentation [6]. Between 2011 and 2015, the number of labiaplasty rates climbed from 2,141 to 8,745, indicating a fourfold increase [6]. Similar increases in procedures over the period from 2001 to 2016 are documented in the UK, Canada, Europe, Australia, India, Brazil and parts of Asia. Numbers of government-subsidised procedures can be accessed from government data in Australia and the UK; however, these represent the tip of the iceberg, as the majority are performed in the private sector. UK government-subsidised procedures indicate FGCS requests increased fivefold for the period 2001–2011, from 397 to 1,726 [7]. The threefold climb in Australia over the 10 years 2003–2013 prompted a review, with subsequent restriction criteria for labiaplasty in 2015. This resulted in a 28% decline in requests through the public sector within one year [8]. The average age range of women requesting labiaplasty is between 25 and 45 years; however, statistics in Australia and the UK indicate that girls and young women from 15 to 24 years of age are presenting with concerns about their genital appearance as frequently as the 25- to 45-year-old age group and that as many as one-third of requests received by GPs in Australia have been from girls under the age of 18 [9].

What Is Normal?

The question often posed to the GP is, "Am I normal down there?" The obvious answer is that 'normal', as with all other physical attributes, covers a wide spectrum and that it is 'normal' to have labia minora that protrude beyond the labia majora in as many as 30%–50% of women. The current classification systems used to measure labia minora classify the common occurrence of labia minora that extend beyond the labia majora along the spectrum of 'labial hypertrophy', thereby reclassifying normal as an abnormal variant warranting surgery. Genital changes can occur with age, parity, hormones, skin disease processes and weight fluctuations [3]. It is important that the doctor informs women and girls that labia minora grow during puberty until full adult maturation is achieved, which is around 18 years and that many may have asymmetrical labia minora. Following menopause, labia minora can atrophy and decrease in size.

Issues for the GP

Genital Anatomy Anxiety

A GP will deal with genital anatomy anxiety far more commonly than with requests for labiaplasty [9]. However, if genital normality concerns are not adequately addressed by the GP, women are more likely to explore labiaplasty as a 'correction' towards the 'single slit', due to the normalisation of this being embedded through societal reinforcement [10]. Women and girls who seek information online using the commonly known terms such as 'Barbie-plasty', 'vaginal rejuvenation', 'labiaplasty' and 'designer vagina' are directed to a plethora of commercial websites which promote specific practitioner expertise, many displaying before-and-after photographs. The medicalisation of non-medical conditions on these sites, using terminology which is mostly unknown to the rest of the medical profession, can mislead women and heighten 'genital anxiety'. The marketing strategies can sway emotionally vulnerable women into believing that these 'medical conditions' can be 'corrected' easily, without providing the assurance that the wide variations in appearance are normal [11].

The GP who is aware of these issues has the opportunity to allay genital anatomy concerns, while exploring reasons for the patient's motivation and expectation of outcomes. Recent research indicates that women who are considering labiaplasty and are given time to think about their decision after being shown images depicting the wide range of diversity preoperatively, choose to undergo surgery less frequently [12] (Table 12.1).

Table 12.1 Key points for general practitioners

FGCS is a relatively new cosmetic surgical procedure with increased demand internationally.

GPs have an important role in reassuring women about normality and the long term 'unknowns' of FGCS.

GPs see many women of all ages with genital anatomy anxiety asking,

"Am I normal looking down there?"

Women seeking information online receive skewed information which normalises a pre-pubertal appearance.

Genital anatomy does not fully mature until around age 18 in women and cosmetic surgery should be avoided before this age.

Psychosocial Factors Influencing Women

The range of factors influencing women's perception of genital normality is wide and includes factors such as online pornography and 'photo shopped' images of genitals, which present the external appearance as a simple, hairless slit. Genital hair removal, which has become extremely popular, reveals soft, previously unexposed genital skin, increasing its vulnerability to trauma, skin infections, chafing and rubbing. Women should be made aware that vulval skin is delicate and prone to irritation and if the appearance of their external genital region creates concern for them, they should be provided adequate reassurance of the diversity that exists.

The lack of formal education around genital anatomy and function throughout life extends from school curricula all the way through to medical curricula. A consequence of this lack of education is that online images are then accepted as the norm, and an unrealistic perception is established. Opportunities that are open to the GP to educate women regarding genital anatomy arise at the time of cervical screening / PAP (Papanicolaou) test, consultations around sexually transmitted infection screening (STI screening), contraceptive advice, insertion of intrauterine contraceptive device (IUCD), postpartum (after childbirth) checks and during menopause discussions.

Rapid Increase in Requests Precedes Adequate Education of the Profession

In 1995 the GP population would have had little or no idea regarding the FGCS group of procedures. By 2015, almost all GPs surveyed in a large Australian study were aware of FGCS. Ninety-seven percent had been asked by their female patients about the normality of genital appearance and around 50% had been asked directly for a referral to have labiaplasty surgery [9]. In the UK, this has been referred to as the 'new dilemma for GPs' [1]. The Royal Australian College of General Practitioners (RACGP) responded to the need for professional guidance in dealing with the increase in requests, by developing a guide entitled, 'Female genital cosmetic surgery: A resource for general practitioners and other health professionals' [13]. This is a useful resource and can be downloaded from the RACGP website. Position statements from American College of Obstetricians and Gynecologists (ACOG) [14], Royal College of Obstetricians and Gynaecologists (RCOG)

[15], Society of Obstetricians and Gynaecologists Canada (SOGC) [16], Royal Australian and New Zealand College of Obstetricians and Gynaecologists (RANZCOG)[17] and British Society of Paediatric and Adolescent Gynaecologists (BritSPAG) [18] have also issued guidelines for the health profession (see Resources in the appendix).

Helping a Woman Make an Informed Choice

Adopting the stance that FGCS represents a simple case of women choosing to do with their bodies as they wish neglects to address the background of genital anatomy ignorance endemic among the wider population including health professionals, upon which FGCS has flourished [19]. The doctor is in a unique position to determine whether the patient's concern is due to functional, aesthetic, psychological or a combination of these reasons. The observations should then drive the consultation, including inquiries into any mental health history and any relationship difficulties and/or partner abuse. Although a referral for psychological counselling prior to surgery is often recommended [15], it is not for rubber stamping an intervention that the patient has already signed up to. The purpose of any psychological counselling must be clear. It usually involves a desire for a psychological outcome and the patient must be able to opt in. Although labiaplasty appears to positively elevate women's genital appearance satisfaction, it has not been proven to improve the woman's general psychological well-being or the quality of her intimate relationships or long-term sexual and aesthetic satisfaction outcomes [12].

Common Patient Presentations

The GP needs to be equipped to support patients with a broad range of issues, as demonstrated by the case studies that follow. Table 12.2 summarises the guidance suggested.

Useful Open-ended Questions

How much do you know about your genital anatomy, e.g., the names of the different parts?

What kind of conversations have you had about this? With whom?

CASE STUDY 12.1 An Adolescent Requesting Genital Surgery

Casey, aged 16, presents with her mother. The mother initially starts the conversation by stating that they had made an appointment to see a plastic surgeon for Casey. The mother states, "Her vagina doesn't look right." Casey just had her first Brazilian wax and "Everything is hanging out. It certainly looks different from mine!" Casey is looking unhappy and lets her mother do the talking. The GP asks Casey, "So Casey, what is it that you're feeling?" Casey responds with "I hate it! It's disgusting. It's all just hanging out and I want it cut off!" The GP asks to examine Casey and she consents. Casey is now on the examination couch with the curtain drawn around her and the GP, with the mother still in the room. The GP asks, "So Casey, can you tell me what it is that you don't think is right? What is it that you want cut off?" The GP offers her a mirror to show you what it is that she cannot accept, but Casey refuses to look at herself, so the mirror is put away. Casey has difficulty touching her genital region to demonstrate what exactly she struggles with. She allows the doctor to identify the areas and when they point to her labia minora, she states, "That's the bit. I hate it. I just want a straight line. I don't want these hanging out bits. It's disgusting!" she repeats emphatically. The GP assures both Casey and mother that Casey's vulva is normal and healthy and that the labia minora, often called the vagina lips, often extend beyond the margin of the outer labia. The GP assures Casey and her mother that they will not brush off their concerns. They invite Casey to discuss this further with her mother outside the room, although she can choose to invite her mother back in the room.

Table 12.2 A six-point guide for GPs

1. FGCS incidence is climbing. Informed doctors can reduce unnecessary anxiety regarding vulval genital anatomy, thereby deflecting an increase in FGCS.

2. Patient examination should be performed by the GP or the patient referred to a doctor experienced in women's health. It is an opportunity to educate patients about genital anatomy.

3. Mental health and relationship abuse issues need to be considered and referred for counselling accordingly.

4. Educate patients about genital diversity – use online tools such as www.labialibrary.org Warn patients regarding known and unknown risks of surgery.

5. It is recommended for GPs to refer for gynaecological assessment, in those wishing to have FGCS (in Australia only)

6. Patients younger than 18 should be referred to a psychologist/psychiatrist and specialist adolescent gynaecologist. Surgery should be delayed until genital maturity is achieved.

Modified, courtesy RACGP.

You are unhappy about how your genitals look. In what way are these feelings affecting you, for example, in school work, your friendships?

What about relationships, or sexual activities – what can you tell me about how your feelings affect these aspects of your life?

Tell me, what's going well in your life at the moment?

What's going less well?

As a doctor, I have quite a lot of information to share with you. Is now a good time?

Key Management Considerations

Listen to the Patient

It is good practice to offer Casey the opportunity to be alone with you to talk more about her own concerns, and politely request that the mother wait in the waiting room. This gives Casey the opportunity to express herself without the mother/guardian present and assists in building trust with the GP, not only in this context but for future medical concerns she might have.

Educate the Mother and the Patient

The mother and Casey refer to the whole area as 'the vagina' but they are really referring to the labia minora. This is an opportunity for the GP to educate both the mother and daughter on the correct terminology and the anatomy of the vulva using a simple sketch diagram. This is also an opportune time to refer them to an online site such as the *Labia Library* (www.labialibrary.org.au) [20], or to show them images from a book titled *Femalia* [21], that will allow both mother and daughter to see that the range of diversity is vast and that Casey fits well within the spectrum (see Resources in the appendix). They should be informed that genital development in adolescence reaches completion at around the age of 18 years. It is important to emphasise to Casey and her mother that surgery prior to this time might not result in the outcome expected.

Explore Psychosocial Influences

Casey's choice of language is very strong, as is her expression of repulsion, which should invite further questions regarding how this is affecting her. Is it affecting her ability to do things like swimming and other sports or to be with friends? Ask her how or why she derived this notion that she had a problem. How often does she think about this and how does she feel overall? Is it affecting her ability to sleep or eat and is she avoiding people because of this? Of particular interest is the observation that Casey rejected the offer to look at herself in a mirror during the examination and also refused to touch her genital region to show the GP what it is that she 'hates'. This level of self-disgust should alert the GP to deeper psychosocial issues and warrants further exploration.

Peer pressure is at its most impactful during these years of change and adjustment and there is peer pressure to look, dress and even behave in particular ways. The need for social acceptance can underlie many insecurities surrounding physical appearance, as this is a period during which body image sensitivity, eating disorders, anxiety around acceptance and physical appearance can be heightened.

Refer to a Mental Health Professional

A physical examination should be offered and conducted in the presence of a chaperone. Where there are psychosocial difficulties such as teasing, bullying and body image problems, offer to refer to a psychologist for help. Many of the adolescents requesting surgery have not yet had sexual relations, but fear that they will be undesirable or unable to attract a partner with their particular physical appearance. Where more significant mental health issues are identifiable, e.g., symptoms of body dysmorphic

disorder, eating disorders, self-harm and suicidal ideation, offer to refer to a psychiatrist.

Body dysmorphic disorder (BDD), in the *Diagnostic and Statistical Manual of Mental Disorders*, Fifth Edition (DSM–V) Obsessive–Compulsive Disorders group, can present during adolescence and can continue into adult life. It can develop as a result of teasing, and patients develop an obsessive preoccupation with an aspect of their appearance that they dislike because they believe it is defective and become fixated on it. They see their 'defects' as real, obvious and very severe. They perform repetitive behaviours such as thinking or worrying about their appearance repeatedly throughout the day or for more than 1 hour per day. They might stop socialising, and disruption of daily activities occurs as a direct result of these appearance concerns. The preoccupation is not better accounted for by another mental disorder (e.g., dissatisfaction with body shape and size, as in anorexia nervosa). People with BDD suffer high post-surgery dissatisfaction rates.

Refer to Specialist Adolescent and Paediatric Gynaecologist

As the mother has already made an appointment for Casey to see a plastic surgeon, she should be advised that the current BritSPAG /RCOG guidelines recommend that Casey should be referred to a specialist adolescent and paediatric gynaecologist in the first instance alongside a referral for psychiatric counselling [18]. A team care approach that involves the GP, the counsellor, the gynaecologist and the parent is recommended (Table 12.2).

Another aspect to consider is that genital surgery for aesthetic or functional reasons raises ethical issues for the medical profession, as the removal of genital tissue of any amount falls under the definition of female genital mutilation and as such, begs the question regarding the appropriateness of performing elective surgery which is similar to female

---

CASE STUDY 12.2 An Adult Woman Presents with Labial Discomfort during Exercise

Susan presents stating: "I'm getting a lot of irritation and sometimes I have pain around my vagina. I'm training for my triathlon and I keep getting sore lips that feel hot and sometimes swell, especially when I cycle. It's affecting my ability to perform and I'm really fed up. I mentioned this to a friend in our spin cycle class and she brought up 'labiaplasty' or something like that. I googled it and all these sites came up talking about 'designer vagina' surgery. I want to get this problem fixed and wonder what you know about this type of surgery and whether I should have it."

genital mutilation, in the context of newly evolving cultural and social values [22].

Useful Questions

What sort of exercise gear do you wear?

Did you know that a lot of irritation is caused by G-strings?

Have you tried adjusting your bicycle seat?

Do you wear any padding when you cycle?

When did the irritation start? Was it with increased training or has this always been the case?

Do you remove your pubic hair? If so, what technique do you use?

Do you have a partner and is there any discomfort with sexual intercourse?

How is your relationship going?

How do you feel about your genital appearance?

How is this impacting your life and relationships?

What do you know about the function of the genital tissue?

Key Management Considerations

Provide Practical Solutions for Functional Problems

Susan has presented for advice from her GP, whom she trusts as a source of information. The GP should be aware of FGCS surgery options including short-term

and long-term risks. It is important to point out that labiaplasty is an irreversible procedure for symptoms that might be resolved by modification of clothing and bicycle seat padding or adjustment.

Fashion such as tight clothes, especially exercise apparel that outlines body contour, can emphasise the genital area in women with larger labia. Cycling gear, bike riding, yoga pants, running in tight clothing with G-strings or tight-fitting, small undergarments often cause discomfort and labia can get caught in them. Even sitting on these can be painful such that there is swelling and chafing by the end of the day. The garment is the cause of the presenting problems in most cases, not the underlying anatomy. Choices need to be made by the woman eventually regarding her preference for certain items of clothing, and it is important to emphasise that fashions change; however, surgery is irreversible and might not yield the results desired.

Discuss genital hair removal, as this can increase vulnerability to trauma, skin infections, chafing and rubbing. Shaving, waxing and the more permanent laser hair removal are used on average monthly, and each technique can result in skin irritation. The use of scented products around the genital area should be discouraged, as they can cause or exacerbate dermatitis.

Examine the Patient

In a setting where there is recurrent genital irritation, it is important to examine the genital area to exclude sexually transmitted infections or underlying urogenital skin disease that requires specialist dermatological treatment.

CASE STUDY 12.3 An Adult Woman Presents with Concerns after Childbirth

Anne visits your rooms for her routine Pap smear. She has had her third child, who is now 2, and comments, "I'm dreading this, I hate having Pap smears … since having had kids, things down there aren't quite the same … my husband says I feel loose."

CASE STUDY 12.4 A Postmenopausal Woman Presents with Discomfort during Intercourse

Ingrid is a 58-year-old postmenopausal woman who admits to you during an uncomfortable Pap smear examination that she has had painful intercourse for several years now. The doctor opens up the discussion by commenting, "The Pap smear was very uncomfortable for you today. Do you feel any discomfort like this when you have sex?" She answers, "I avoid sex, doctor. It's too uncomfortable. I feel very dry and it hurts when he enters." Regarding treatment options you offer her, she states, "I don't want any hormones, doctor. I'm worried about the breast cancer side of things." She goes on to say, "I heard about this laser treatment called 'vaginal rejuvenation' or something … does it work, doctor?"

Risks of Surgery

The discussion with the doctor should include the uncertainty of outcomes of surgery and options for managing functional symptoms where they exist. Explanation needs to include the known short-term risks of FGCS such as bleeding, wound dehiscence, infection and scarring along the outer edge of the labia, which can disrupt the neurovascular supply and affect sexual sensation. Other complications can include dyspareunia, removal of too much tissue resulting in exposure of the clitoris to clothing causing chronic pain, reduced or altered sexual sensitivity, scar retraction and nodularity. Assessment of the presenting concern by the patient should be combined with documentation of a baseline psychosexual history, culminating in examination and education of the patient.

Useful Questions

How are things at home?

How are things between you and your husband?

What sort of things has he said to you?

How did that make you feel when he said that?

How has your sex life changed for you?

Is sex uncomfortable? Do you enjoy sex?

You say things feel different during sex. What does that that mean?

Do you have any leakage of urine when you sneeze, cough or laugh?

Key Management Considerations

Relationship Issues and Counselling

Ask Anne if there is marital disharmony or partner pressure to look a particular way. Referral for relationship counselling will be more helpful than a referral for surgery. In different settings, a woman who is in a new relationship after a long-term destructive one has ended might feel a need to 'renew herself' and counselling is warranted in this setting also. It is important to inquire about past sexual abuse issues or domestic violence which might underlie the desire to change her appearance. Her concern about genital anatomy might be affecting her sexual confidence and there might be avoidance of sexual relations due to this which might in turn affect her relationship [23]. Screening for depression and anxiety which can result from these consequences is important.

Examination and Appropriate Referral to Allied Health

During and following the postpartum period the woman might be concerned regarding changes related to vaginal delivery such as vaginal laxity, stress urinary incontinence and pelvic organ prolapse. The postpartum check should include discussion concerning these symptoms and a referral for expert pelvic floor and continence physiotherapy should be recommended for pregnancy- and birth-related changes. Review of symptoms following a set course of sessions should assess the level of improvement, and where dissatisfaction persists, referral to a gynaecologist or urogynaecologist might be necessary.

Useful Questions

Do you use any lubrication with intercourse? Has this made a difference?

Is sex painful? Has it always been painful or has this been since you reached menopause?

Can you achieve orgasm and has this changed?

Do you have any trouble with your bladder?

Does it hurt when you pass urine? Do you feel you need to go all the time?

What other symptoms do you have?

Key Management Considerations

Urogenital Syndrome of Menopause

Vaginal atrophy is a significant problem that affects between 25% and 50% of post-menopausal women within 5 years of menopause. It often presents in the perimenopausal phase, and unlike hot flushes, tends not to diminish with age. It can also occur in women who have had premature or surgical menopause for cancer prevention or treatment. Symptoms that arise from the reduction of oestrogen can include painful intercourse (superficial dyspareunia), vaginal dryness, altered or unpleasant sensation (dysaethesia), slower or diminished sexual arousal, anorgasmia, bladder dysfunction such as urinary frequency, recurrent urinary tract infections and stress urinary incontinence. The physiological way to preserve vaginal and bladder function is through oestrogenisation with low doses of intravaginal oestrogen, with or without systemic oral hormone replacement therapy. In situations where there is a history of breast or gynaecological cancer, women might prefer to avoid even low-dose intravaginal oestrogen. Other options include non-hormonal vaginal moisturisers and lubricating jellies.

Treatment Options When Hormone Replacement Therapy Is Not Enough or Not Desired

There are occasions on which a patient will refuse to, or cannot have topical oestrogen therapy but still requires treatment of this complex suite of symptoms, and to date, very little else has been available. The MonaLisa Touch® is a fractionated CO_2 laser developed by DEKA which has been tested at the University of Milan as an alternative to oestrogen therapy specifically for post-cancer patients, and was rapidly taken to market for the treatment of post-menopausal urogenital syndrome, without larger trials being conducted. The pinpoint laser beams are delivered through a wand-like instrument which has a multitude of tiny perforations on its surface and is inserted into the vagina. Multiple dot-like areas receive a thermal injury over a 10-minute session, which over several treatments has been shown in some small studies to regenerate collagen and blood vessels. The premise behind the development of this tool is that similar CO_2 fractionated laser treatments have already been approved for use on the face with good results when used by trained specialists. Currently, fractionated CO_2 has not been widely approved for use for the urogenital symptoms associated with menopause, as the studies published are small and despite their favourable outcomes, concern exists that unregulated use might result in scarring or worsen symptoms if patients are not carefully examined to rule out urogenital disease other than atrophy, including sexually transmitted infections, and if adequate training is not received.

Medical Entrepreneurialism and Opportunism

Much of the online marketing of such laser procedures associates 'vaginal rejuvenation' as a return to genital 'youth' post birth, or post menopause. The surgical option for 'vaginal rejuvenation' is usually performed to correct post birth vaginal laxity, sometimes in conjunction with surgery for stress urinary incontinence or pelvic organ prolapse. Criteria exist for the surgical suite of treatments but

are lacking for the treatment of urogenital symptoms with laser. An inexperienced person might overlook genital tract disease, infection and even cause laser burns to the genital tract. Laser for vaginal atrophy has not been approved by RCOG, ACOG and RANZCOG as yet, and the outcomes of the larger clinical trials currently being conducted in several countries will inform physician guidelines in due course. Entrepreneurialism in medicine is often not rewarded by the profession but by the commercial world; however, our duty is to provide care for patients and to do no harm and wait until we can confidently mitigate the short- and long-term harmful effects.

The Examination and Basic Anatomy

Examine the patient respectfully and provide education regarding genital anatomy function and diversity with confidence. It is helpful to provide the patient with a mirror at the time of examination. An understanding of genital anatomy is required by the doctor in order to assist the patient in understanding the anatomy and function of the various, mostly hidden structures (see Chapter 2). The diagrams in Figure 12.1 provide a good basis for discussion and can be used to explain the names and functions of the vulva, which includes the vaginal opening, the urethra, clitoris, labia majora, the labia minora and mons pubis. It is also important to exclude genital and vulvar skin diseases such as lichen sclerosis, chronic candidiasis, genital warts, vulvar dermatitis, carcinoma, vulvar lymphoedema, trauma related to sex and other genital skin diseases at this time. Sometimes it is not possible to proceed to a physical examination because of patient embarrassment, and a follow-up appointment can be offered alongside the information regarding reputable online information sites (see Resources in the appendix).

In the primary care setting, formal measurements of genital structures are not required, as this might imply that there is a 'normal' measure. The sexual satisfaction scale [24] and the genital appearance assessment scale [23] can help determine the impact the presenting concern is having on the woman as well as uncovering other factors that are at play.

Resources for the Doctor

Helpful resources for the doctor and the patient are listed in the Resources in the appendix. The list is not exhaustive; however, the key resource that currently

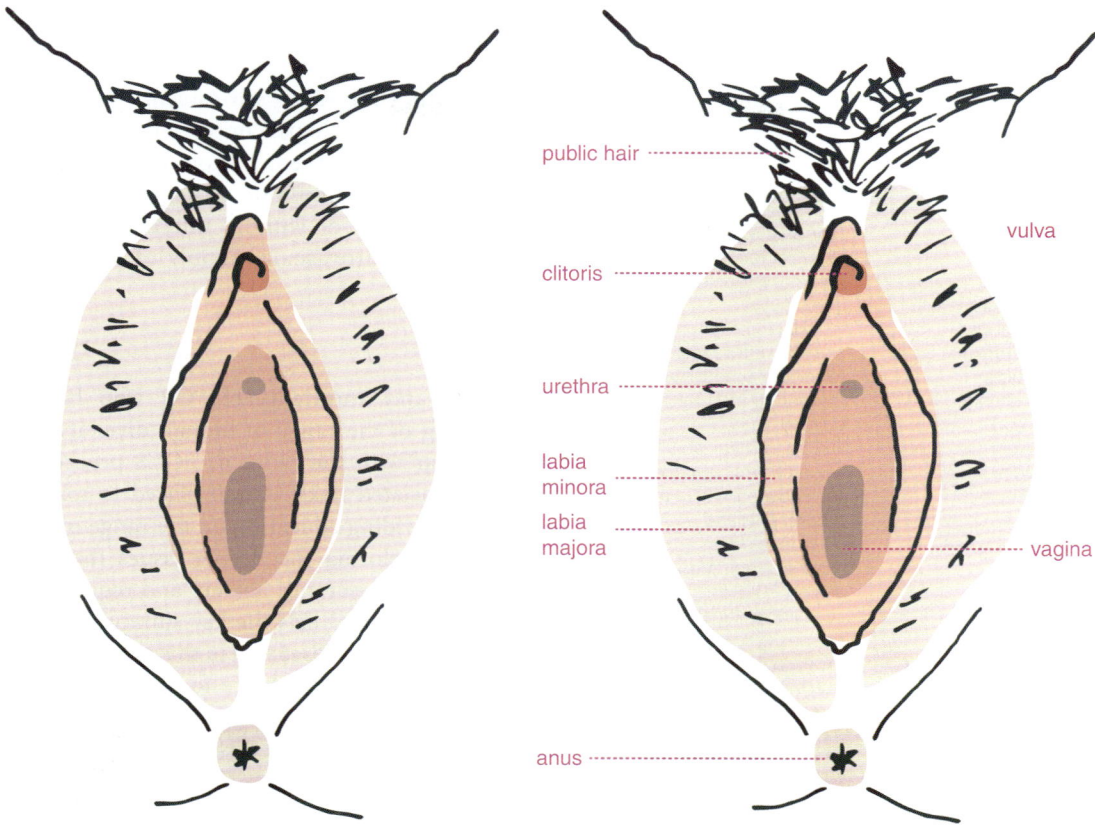

Figure 12.1 **Diagrams for use in the clinical setting.** (Courtesy Women's Health Victoria.)

exists for GPs to date is the RACGP FGCS guide [13]. This provides a sound base upon which the health professional can gain a better understanding of how to take a history, perform an examination and address the issues.

What Women Who Decide to Have Surgery Should Be Aware of

When a woman makes a request for referral for FGCS following consultation with the GP, she should bear in mind that perceptions of normality vary significantly across the different medical specialties, and even the gender of the doctor [25]. There are several different surgical approaches and there are no set criteria determining which should be adopted on a patient-by-patient basis, so a woman should know what outcome she seeks and clearly stipulate this. FGCS can be performed by any practitioner with a medical degree ranging from gynaecologists, plastic surgeons, cosmetic surgeons, urologists, urogynaecologists and

GPs with minimal or no training in the procedure. There are no standard guidelines for labiaplasty, and it is performed based mostly on women's dissatisfaction with their labia [11].

Women may undertake surgery in the belief that it will enhance their genital appearance, improve their sex life and elevate their self-confidence. None of these can be guaranteed [12]. An Australian study revealed that serious adverse events at the time of admission or requiring readmission within 2 weeks of the initial procedure occurred in around 7% of procedures and 4% of the patients had repeat procedures [26]. Caesarean section rates were 30% higher in these women, presumably due to planned birth interventions although birth-related perineal trauma due to previous FGCS appeared not to increase [26]. Although the majority of surgeons report as high as up to 95% patient satisfaction with the surgical outcome, these claims do not demonstrate post-surgery sexual satisfaction scales and long-term genital appearance satisfaction (Chapter 6). Women must be made

Table 12.3 Summary points

Current status	Recommendations
• Genital anatomy anxiety is common. • Women and girls have poor knowledge around genital anatomy, anatomical names, function and diversity. • Genital anatomy education is lacking from all medical and non-medical curricula. • FGCS rise reflects sociocultural change. • Adolescents and younger women are particularly vulnerable. • Long-term effects of FGCS on sexual function are unknown.	• Assess degree of anxiety and manage accordingly. Education provides comfort for patients. • Provide education tools that explain function, names and diversity of genital anatomy. • Introduce genital anatomy education from early schooling, through to medical training. • FGCS and medical opportunism need to be regulated. • Adolescents and younger women should be advised against FGCS for aesthetic or functional reasons. A second expert opinion and psychological assessment are required. • Studies reveal that more genital surface area is associated with increased sexual pleasure and responsiveness. Inform women of this.

aware that the sensorineural function of the genital tissue that is removed is not properly understood. It is assumed the removed tissue is redundant without clinical evidence to support this. The labia minora is second to the clitoris in terms of sexual nerve innervation, provides lubrication during sexual arousal and changes in size and shape throughout life [24].

Post-surgery Follow-up

Genital self-image is an important component of one's overall health and quality of life [27]. Keeping this in mind, women who elect to have an FGCS procedure should be followed up by their GP post-surgery, as with all other surgical procedures. Arrange an appointment to gauge the short-term and long-term effects and document these. If the outcome is not satisfactory, the woman might feel embarrassed to admit this, so it is important to observe non-verbal cues when asking

and offer support. The woman might be considering revision surgery to remove more tissue, or she might be experiencing painful intercourse and subsequent relationship and self-esteem difficulties. Referral to a psychologist or sex therapist and review with her surgeon should be offered. Sometimes, a second opinion is required if there is chronic pain with or without intercourse due to damage to the neurovascular supply of the genital area.

Summary

A confident and knowledgeable GP who has an understanding of the range of human diversity, but is also familiar with the range of FGCS procedures and their associated risks, is well placed to manage patients by providing education on the range of normality while exploring the deeper issues that may underlie genital appearance anxiety and requests for vulvoplasty. Table 12.3 lists the key summary points and recommendations discussed in this chapter. A full list of key professional guidance for medical practitioners and other useful materials can be found in the Resources in the appendix of this book.

References

1. Liao LM, Creighton SM. Female genital cosmetic surgery: A new dilemma for GPs. *Br J Gen Pract*. 2011;61:7–8

2. Reitsma W, Mourits MJE, Koning M, Pascal A, van der Lei B. No (wo)man is an island: The influence of physicians' personal predisposition to labia minora appearance on their clinical decision making: A cross-sectional survey. *J Sex Med*. 2011;8(8):2377–85.

3. Bramwell R, Morland C. Genital appearance satisfaction in women: The development of a questionnaire and exploration of correlates. *J Reprod Infant Psychol*. 2009;**27**:15–27. doi:10.1080/02646830701759793.

4. Braun V. In search of (better) sexual pleasure: Female genital "cosmetic" surgery. *Sexualities*. 2005;8:407–24.

5. Goodman MP. Female cosmetic genital surgery. *Obstet Gynecol*. 2009;113(1):154–9.

6. American Society for Aesthetic Plastic Surgery. ASAPS statistics, 2016. Available from: www.surgery.org/media/statistics

7. Crouch NS, Deans R, Michala L, Liao LM, Creighton SM. Clinical characteristics of well women seeking labial reduction surgery: A prospective study. *BJOG*. 2011;118, 1507–10. doi:10.1111/j.1471–0528.2011.03088.x.

8. Australian Government Department of Human Services. Medicare Item Reports. Available from: http://medicarestatistics.humanservices.gov.au/statistics/mbs_item.jsp.

9. Simonis M, Manocha R, Ong J. Female genital cosmetic surgery: A cross-sectional survey exploring knowledge, attitude and practice of general practitioners. *BMJOpen*. 2016;6(9). Available from: http://dx.doi.org/10.1136/bmjopen-2016–013010

10. Sharp G, Tiggemann M, Mattiske J. Predictors of consideration of labiaplasty: An extension of the tripartite influence model of beauty ideals. *Psychol Women Q*.11 September 2014. Available from: http://pwq.sagepub.com/content/early/2014/09/11/0361684314549949

11. Clinch NC, Osland A, Wang C. Legitimizing radical new medical services. *J Appl Business Econ*. 2011;12 (4):67–78.

12. Sharp G, Tiggemann M, Mattiske J. Psychological outcomes of labiaplasty: A prospective study. *Plast Reconstruct Surg*. 2016; 138(6):1202–9. doi: 10.1097/PRS.0000000000002751.

13. Royal Australian College of General Practitioners. Female genital cosmetic surgery: A resource for general practitioners and other health professionals, 2015. Available from: www.racgp.org.au/your-practice/guidelines/female-genital-cosmetic-surgery/

14. Committee on Adolescent Health Care, American College of Obstetricians and Gynecologists. ACOG Committee Opinion No. 662: Breast and labial surgery in adolescents. *Obstet Gynecol*. 2016;127:e138–e140.

15. RCOG/BritSPAG: Royal College of Obstetricians and Gynaecologists and British Society for Paediatric and Adolescent Gynaecology. Joint RCOG/BritSPAG release: Issues surrounding women and girls undergoing female genital cosmetic surgery explored. Available from: www.rcog.org.uk/en/news/joint-rcog-britspag-release-issues-surrounding-women-and-girls-undergoing-female-genital-cosmetic-surgery-explored

16. Society of Obstetricians and Gynaecologists of Canada. SOGC Policy No. 300 December 2013. Female genital cosmetic surgery. Available from: https://sogc.org/wp-content/uploads/2013/09/December2013-CPG300-ENG-Online_final.pdf. Shaw D, Lefebvre G, Bouchard C, et al. Female genital cosmetic surgery. *J Obstet Gynaecol Can*. 2013;35(12):1108–14.

17. RANZCOG. Vaginal 'rejuvenation' and cosmetic vaginal procedures C-Gyn 24, First endorsed by RANZCOG: July 2008 Current: March 2015, Amended July 2016. Available from: www.ranzcog.edu.au/RANZCOG_SITE/media/RANZCOG-MEDIA/Women's%20Health/Statement%20and%20guidelines/Clinical%20-%20Gynaecology/Vaginal-rejuvenation,-laser-and-cosmetic-procedures-%28C-Gyn-24%29-Amended-July-2016.pdf?ext=.pdf

18. British Society for Paediatric and Adolescent Gynaecology Position Statement: Labial Reduction Surgery (Labiaplasty) on Adolescents, October 2013. Available from: www.britspag.org/sites/default/files/downloads/Labiaplasty final Position Statement.pdf

19. Andrikopoulou M, Michala L, Creighton SM, Liao LM. The normal vulva in medical textbooks. *J Obst Gynaecol*. 2013;33(7):648–50.

20. Labia Library. www.labialibrary.org.au

21. Blank J, ed. *Femalia*. San Francisco: Last Gasp; 2011.

22. Cain JM, Iglesia CB, Dickens B, Montgomery O. Body enhancement through female genital cosmetic surgery creates ethical and rights dilemmas. *Int J Gynaecol Obstet*. 2013;122:169–72.

23. Schick VR, Calabrese SK, Rima BN, Zucker AN. Genital appearance dissatisfaction: Implications for women's genital image self-consciousness, sexual esteem, sexual satisfaction, and sexual risk. *Psychol Women Q*. 2010;34:394–404. doi:10.1111/j.1471–6402.2010.01584.x.

24. Schober JM, Alguacil NM, Cooper RS, Pfaff DW, Meyer-Bahlburg HFL. Self-assessment of anatomy, sexual sensitivity, and function of the labia and vagina. *Clin Anat*. 2015;28 (3):355–62. doi:10.1002/ca.22503.

25. Braun V, Wilkinson S. Socio-cultural representations of the vagina. *J Reprod Infant Psychol*. 2001;19 (1):17–32.

26. Ampt AJ, Roach V, Roberts CL. Vulvoplasty in New South Wales, 2001–2013: A population-based record linkage study. *Med J Aust*. 2016;205(8):365–9. doi: 10.5694/mja16.00512.

27. Berman LA, Berman J, Miles M, et al. Genital self-image as a component of sexual health: Relationship between genital self-image, female sexual function, and quality of life measures. *J Sex Marital Ther*. 2003;29:11–21.

Female Genital Cosmetic Surgery
Psychological Aspects and Approaches

Lori A. Brotto, Maggie Bryce and Nicole Todd

Background: Women and Cosmetic Surgery

According to the 2016 report of the American Society of Plastic Surgeons [1], the number of people seeking cosmetic surgery continues to rise, with an increase of 3% from the previous year. The majority (92%) of the consumers were women. This amounted to a total of 17.1 million cosmetic surgeries performed in the United States. Breast augmentation remains the most popular and common cosmetic procedure, with more than 290,000 American women receiving breast enhancement in 2016, up 4% from 2015 and up 37% since the year 2000.

Empirical research on psychological factors in the uptake of breast augmentation is sparse. Some research has studied background psychological and personality characteristics. A review of 65 studies found that in general, women who sought cosmetic surgery were more likely to have a narcissistic personality (25% of those seeking surgery vs. 1% of the general population) defined by an unexplained grandiosity and need for admiration [2]. The review also found those seeking cosmetic procedures are more likely (10% of the patients vs. 1.8% of the general population) to have a histrionic personality, defined in terms of attention-seeking behaviour and extreme emotionality.

Women seeking breast augmentation are more likely to be Caucasian, in the age range of 20s to mid-40s, thin and tall, well educated, and have a higher likelihood of a history of depression and anxiety [3]. They are also more likely to be a smoker, to regularly consume alcohol, and to have had a psychiatric hospital admission in the past [3]. A study by Moser and Aiken [4] applied the Theory of Planned Behaviour to explore intentions for seeking breast augmentation, from both positive and negative cognitive and emotional perspectives. Through a combination of 11 focus groups and subsequent questionnaires administered to 400 women who were considering breast augmentation, they found that women's intentions were significantly predicted by anticipated regret (i.e., women expecting to regret the surgery were less likely to seek surgery), and subjective norms and attitudes (i.e., women attuned to the approval from others were more likely to seek surgery). Women's indirect attitudes, such as expectations for better self-image, enhanced sex appeal, and better perceived appearance were associated with lower levels of anticipated regret over having the breast augmentation. The findings from this study suggest that psychosocial factors can predict cosmetic surgery uptake and outcome. Psychosocial research could therefore usefully inform psychological assessment and interventions.

Psychological Factors and Female Genital Cosmetic Surgery

Although female genital cosmetic surgery (FGCS) was not among the top five most popular cosmetic surgeries in the 2016 report of the American Society of Plastic Surgeons [1], it was notable that FGCS was up 39% in 2016 from 2015, an increase that was greater than in every other type of cosmetic surgery. Though systematic reviews have yet to be conducted on the characteristics of women seeking FGCS, insights into personality types and motives for surgery may be drawn from the literature examining other individuals who seek cosmetic procedures. Some argue that women seeking breast augmentation share similar traits to women seeking FGCS given that both entail alteration to parts of the body associated with female sexuality, although the surgical procedures are clearly different, with different possible complications. Indeed, among women seeking FGCS, previous breast augmentation was the most common prior cosmetic procedure obtained by this group [5].

Among the different types of FGCS, labiaplasty, or surgical alteration to the labia majora and minora, has become the most popular surgery, founded on widespread denigration of female genitalia. Often described as a passive receptacle for the penis, female genitals have been depicted as disgusting, sexually inadequate, vulnerable/abused and even dangerous [6]. The problem-saturated views of female genitalia have undoubtedly impacted on how women view female genitals including their own [6]. A study with young adult women showed a clear relationship between women's perceptions of female genitalia and their own genital self-perceptions [7].

Anxiety associated with perceived vulvar anomalies has undoubtedly increased over recent decades. Hairless, undefined vulvas that have no protruding labia minora have been increasingly emphasised in Western culture and media [8–10]. Women have become more self-conscious of their genitals as a result of these depictions [3,11,12]. Pubic hair removal has thus become popular if not normative and further draws attention to vulvar appearance details [13], in private and public spaces (e.g., communal showers). Women's preference and perception of 'normal' is now the 'Barbie doll ideal' [8]. For example, women will rate vulvar images as more 'normal' and 'representative of society's ideal' with digital and surgical modifications [14].

In reality, the notion of 'normal' is a fallacy given that, like snowflakes, no two vulvas look the same. Their size, shape, texture and colour vary enormously; these variations are not reliably predicted by differences in ethnicity, hormone use, sexual history and other personal and demographic dimensions [15]. Sexualising media have helped to construct a 'designer vulva' that minimises naturally occurring normal variations [16].

Given the subjectivity in the perception of what is 'normal' when it comes to vulvar appearance, there is a critical need to consider the key role for psychological factors in women's genital self-perceptions, dissatisfaction and the desire for cosmetic alteration. However, the literature on psychological predictors of FGCS is not only sparse, but biased, owing to the expectancy of patients and the surgeon carrying out costly assessments. For example, women may downplay any negative or judgemental attitudes that could be perceived as contributing to their requests. Among the existing studies that have examined psychological characteristics of women seeking FGCS, there is evidence for the influence of personal negative judgements and evaluations, perceived partner-related dissatisfaction and perceived negative evaluations by others. In order to adequately consider each of these domains in the context of a psychosocial assessment of women seeking FGCS, it is important to explore each of these in turn.

Personal Factors

A Google search of 'labiaplasty' in 2018 produced 1.32 million hits. Google analytics keep track of such searches generated by high-risk women, and increase direct-to-consumer marketed advertisements that offer low-cost procedures, feeding the consumer market that thrives off self-conscious women [17–20]. In a general sample of women, self-esteem is significantly and negatively associated with satisfaction with genital appearance, suggesting that women with low self-esteem may be particularly vulnerable to appearance schemas (defined as cognitive structures that organise one's experience and actions related to their appearance) [21], though in another study there were no significant differences in self-esteem between women who were and those who were not seeking FGCS [3]. There is significant pressure on women to meet impossible and unrealistic beauty standards. These findings suggest that women with low self-esteem are especially at risk, leading to a vicious cycle such that women's insecurities about their body lead to more exposure to, and vulnerability of, FGCS practices that promise to quell anxieties and raise satisfaction. Indeed, aesthetic dissatisfaction is the leading reason for seeking FGCS and supersedes functional reasons such as vulvar discomfort or pain [22].

In the only controlled study of women seeking FGCS ($n = 55$) versus those who were not ($n = 70$), the surgery seekers had a lower overall quality of life and body image, although they were no more likely to experience anxiety and depression than the control group [23].

Some women may seek FGCS as a means of improving sexual function. Sexual difficulties affect up to a third of women across ages [24], and psychological factors, such as depression, anxiety and body image, are strong predictors of women's sexual response and satisfaction [25]. Some advertisements for FGCS promise to improve sexual function, and according to a short-term retrospective study conducted by the surgical providers, 92% of their patients and their partners reported satisfaction and improved sexual responses with vaginal tightening and labiaplasty [26]. In the only prospective study to evaluate the effects of FGCS on sexual response, only 18 of the original 33 women evaluated at pre-surgery completed post-surgery measures of sexual function, and even fewer completed the follow-up 6–9 months later [27]. Most measures of sexual response did not significantly change post-FGCS. Thus, whereas sexual satisfaction improved at immediate post-surgery, rates fell back to baseline levels when women were assessed at follow-up.

The lack of a control group and the bias inherent in having the treatment team conducting the assessments means that the reliability of these findings is questionable (see Chapter 6, this volume). Given how common relationship and sexual difficulties and dissatisfaction are for women, including younger women [24,28], the promise of positive sexual outcomes would be a compelling motivation to seek cosmetic genital procedures. However, women are not likely informed that the impact of these surgical procedures on the underlying vascular and neural pathways that contribute to sexual response and pleasure is totally unknown (Chapters 2 and 9, this volume).

In summary, although women may seek FGCS to increase sexual desire and/or improve sexual response, at present there is no evidence to suggest that these expectations are met, especially over the long term. The implications for counselling women seeking FGCS are considered in a later section.

Perceived Partner-Related Dissatisfaction

As a group, women seeking cosmetic labiaplasty are more self-conscious, believe that they are less attractive to their partner, and tend to be less satisfied with their lives overall [3,29]. Being in a relationship seems to buffer somewhat against these negative psychological attributions [3]. Although women seeking labiaplasty are concerned that partners do not find them attractive [29], there is evidence that partners themselves have more favourable views than the women might expect [7]. Given women's distorted views about their partner's perception of their genitals, it can be useful for women who are in relationships to be accompanied by their sexual partner at the pre-surgery assessment. This has the advantage of allowing a clinician to identify partner-related perspectives and to gauge whether outcome expectancy is realistic. In a controlled comparison of one group of women seeking and another not seeking FGCS, there were no group differences in the women's reported relationship satisfaction [3]. The

authors concluded that women are not likely to be seeking FGCS as a means of improving relationship satisfaction. Nonetheless, women may still be having specific worries about a partner's view of her genitals, even if the overall relationship was unproblematic.

Perceived Negative Evaluations by Others

In one of the few studies comparing women seeking FGCS to a control group [3], the influence of media ideals and women's internalisation of those ideals differed quite significantly between groups. Those seeking FGCS were more likely to have seen more media images and expressed a stronger desire to resemble those images. In particular, internet images and exposure to advertisements for FGCS were identified as predictors of wish for FGCS [3]. This replicated findings in other studies [11,30].

Negative evaluation by others or negative comments about female genitals made by others can also impact on female genital self-image. In one study, a third of the women who sought FGCS had experienced negative comments by partners, family members or friends [31]. Bullying behaviour is known to contribute to self-consciousness, poor psychological functioning and increased desire for cosmetic procedures in teenagers [32]. It is therefore especially important that during the consultation, the clinician assesses whether there have been harmful comments by others, and whether these comments were actual, perceived or anticipated.

Body Dysmorphia and Perceptual Distortions

Body dysmorphic disorder (BDD) is a diagnosis in the Fifth Edition of the *Diagnostic and Statistical Manual of Mental Disorders* [33] and characterised by one or more perceived defects of flaws in physical appearance. The perceived flaw may be not observed or observed only minimally by others. Nevertheless, to the person affected, it evokes clinically significant distress or impairment which is associated with compensatory behaviours such as mirror checking, reassurance seeking and/or comparing her appearance to that of others. BDD typically begins in adolescence and can have a chronic course punctuated by remissions and relapses [34]. People with BDD make maladaptive interpretations of their appearance, leading to increased anxiety, depression and unhelpful behaviours [35].

BDD is more prevalent among cosmetic surgery users. Only 2% of the general population meet formal criteria for BDD [34] compared to 18–20% of women requesting labiaplasty, according to some studies [20,23]. This is in line with the 14–24.5% prevalence in people pursuing aesthetic surgery [35]. Although there could be short-term improvement in BDD symptoms, cosmetic surgery does not lead to long-term improvement of BDD symptoms [34,35]. While only a proportion of women seeking FGCS would meet formal diagnostic criteria for BDD, we strongly recommend that BDD is part of a comprehensive psychological assessment before surgery. Guidelines for the psychological assessment of BDD among women seeking FGCS are outlined in a subsequent section.

Gaps in Research on Psychological Factors

The literature is scant when it comes to evaluating the psychological characteristics of women seeking FGCS. Even less is known about the psychological, relational and sexual outcomes of FGCS. More importantly, among the existing studies, this literature suffers from significant methodological limitations. These are outlined in Table 13.1, in which strategies for future research are also suggested.

Role of the Medical Expert

This topic is addressed in detail in Chapter 12 (this volume). Suffice to say that physicians at the point of entry into the medical system play a crucial role in beginning the process of critical psychoeducation for women seeking FGCS [37] influenced by factors such as appearance concerns, physical discomfort, media influence, genital shame and perceived partner expectation [38]. Most women requesting labiaplasty have normative labial dimensions [39]. Visible labia minora are as common as recessed labia minora [40]. The viewing of manipulated vulval images can negatively influence a woman's perception of what she considers normal and desirable [14,41], while viewing of images of natural vulvas can improve genital self-image [42] We strongly recommend that health care providers keep a variety of educational resources in their office setting including, for example, picture books like *Petals* [43], educational websites like the Labia Library [44] and Great Wall of Vagina [45] and videos such as Labiaplasty [46] (see also Resources in the appendix). Surgery should never be offered on the initial consultation and never to teenage girls whose genital development is as yet incomplete [37,39]. Adolescents should be supported in their exploration of identity and self-concept rather than being operated on [20].

Table 13.1 Methodological limitations in research on psychological factors associated with FGCS

Existing limitation	Proposed alternative for future research
Sample sizes tend to be very small.	Studies need to be powered to detect significant differences. Effect sizes, response rates and attrition rates at follow-ups should be reported in all studies.
Studies do not include a comparison group of women with similar demographic profiles.	Demographically matched groups of women not seeking FGCS need to be included.
Retrospective design	Outcomes should be measured before and after surgery and at a future follow-up time point.
Participants are recruited from specialty and/or private clinics that offer FGCS, which may bias outcomes given that women have typically paid expenses out-of-pocket for such procedures, and cognitive dissonance theory, which posits that people seek to have harmony between behaviour (spending money on cosmetic procedures) and beliefs (seeking FGCS is a good thing), is at play.	Recruitment should be broader, from public hospitals and health centres. There is a critical need for future research to take account of cognitive dissonance factors in women's self-reported FGCS outcomes.
Lack of long-term follow-up of women who have received FGCS – there is preliminary evidence that even when there are self-reported improvements after surgery (at least in the domain of sexual satisfaction), these tend to disappear by 9-month follow-up [27].	Women should be assessed in the long-term follow-up.
Regret long after the surgery is not typically measured, yet may impact outcomes.	Together with measuring cognitive dissonance [36], efforts should be made to measure regret.

Role of the Psychological Expert

The probing for pre-existing psychological factors such as poor self-esteem, eating problems and tendencies to anxiety require the skills of a psychological clinician. In our experience, this kind of integrated care is far from typical in the cosmetic surgery industry. Nevertheless, we strongly recommend that every woman seeking FGCS undergoes a comprehensive psychosocial and psychosexual assessment by a qualified mental health expert. The components of this assessment, as outlined in Table 13.2, should include (1) motivations for FGCS; (2) assessment of psychiatric symptoms and diagnoses, including BDD; (3) assessment of body image, self-esteem and genital self-image; (4) sexual and relationship factors, including current sexual response and expectations of change with surgery; and (5) exposure to and influence of media ideals, and associated perceptions of others' evaluations.

Assessing for Body Dysmorphic Disorder

We recommend that the provider carry out a thorough assessment of BDD using the criteria laid out by the DSM-5 [33]. A diagnosis of BDD is a predictor of poorer psychosocial outcomes after cosmetic surgery [47], and effort should therefore be made to screen for BDD in advance. This entails a careful, respectful and Socratic-style questioning of preoccupations with the appearance of the genitals. In some cases, we would recommend the use of a validated assessment of BDD, such as the Body Dysmorphic Disorder Questionnaire [48] which can be used as a screening tool, or the Body Dysmorphic Disorder modification of the Yale–Brown Obsessive–Compulsive Scale [49] as a much more detailed assessment of BDD.

Furthermore, as symptoms of BDD may overlap with symptoms of a social anxiety disorder [33], the latter should also be part of the assessment. Essentially, it is important to decipher whether the woman's fear of being negatively evaluated by a partner or by others is due to her appearance or to a more general fear of being embarrassed.

Psychological Treatment Strategies

Depending on the range and severity of distorted body-related thoughts experienced by the woman seeking FGCS, and by the range and intensity of the

Table 13.2 Outline of a psychosocial and sexual assessment for women seeking FGCS

Motivation for FGCS	Assess for motivations related to perceived physical flaw in genital appearance, concerns about appearing abnormal, physical discomfort and pain. Given that women may be highly motivated to receive FGCS and aware of barriers or difficulties toward that end, women may minimise psychological motivations and emphasise functional ones.
Assessment of psychiatric symptoms and diagnoses, including BDD	A history of anxiety and depression are significant risk factors for poor psychosocial outcomes after cosmetic surgery and must be assessed. This includes history as well as current symptoms of an anxiety disorder and major depressive disorder, as well as subthreshold clinical syndromes. Given that women with BDD are more likely to seek cosmetic surgeries of all types, it is important that the clinician assess for the symptoms of BDD and determine the extent to which perceived distortions of the genitals are contributing to the desire for FGCS.
Assessment of body image, self-esteem, and genital self-image	Assess general attitudes to female genitalia and the individual's perceptions of her own genitals. Ask about her perception of normal and consider showing photos of a range of vulvas during this assessment to gauge reactions on the perception of what is normal. Assess self-esteem by asking questions about the woman's life more generally and her feelings about key aspects of her life.
Sexual and relationship factors, including current sexual response and expectations of change with surgery	Ask about all domains of sexual function: desire, arousal, lubrication, orgasm, sexual satisfaction and sexual pain. Validated measures can also be used. Inquire about the woman's expectations about the impact of FGCS on sexual functioning. If in a relationship, ask about partner's own sexual function, and her perceptions of the partner's view of her sexual functioning. Ask about pressure placed on her by a partner to seek FGCS, and whether this pressure is actual or perceived. If possible, try to assess the partner separately to inquire about the woman's reasons for FGCS. This might also include asking about partner's perceptions of the look of the woman's genitals and what has been expressed.
Exposure to and influence of media ideals, and associated perceptions of others' evaluations	Inquire about exposure to pornography and the woman's attitudes, beliefs and emotions when viewing such images, and how those images might have influenced her wish for FGCS. Assess for negative evaluation by others or negative comments about female genitals made by others. Bullying behaviour is known to contribute to self-consciousness and poor psychological functioning, so that a desire for cosmetic procedures in teenagers should be assessed.

associated emotions, an individualised psychological treatment plan may be required. Ideally, this would be offered as an alternative to FGCS. There is, however, as yet no evidence that psychological interventions can reduce the prevalence of FGCS. In our own experience working within a multidisciplinary team in a large metropolitan centre, however, targeted psychological therapy can prevent or delay surgery in the majority of cases. Even if the woman has already decided on surgery, should there be clear indications for psychological interventions, they could take place post-surgery at some point.

Based on the generic empirical literature for body image concerns and distortions, we recommend individually tailored applications of psycho-therapeutic techniques drawn on: (1) behaviour therapy, (2) cognitive behavioural therapy, (3) mindfulness-based therapy and (4) sex therapy.

Behaviour Therapy

Behaviour therapy focuses on identifying problematic behaviours including avoidance. This type of work focuses on helping people to take a step at a time to distract from, delay, or inhibit performing unhelpful behaviours and on taking up more adaptive new behaviours. A component of behaviour therapy is exposure. This involves the progressive and systematic exposure to what is feared or avoided, in this case an area of the body, that elicits anxiety and shame. By building exposure to the feared object or situation, anxiety will progressively decrease. This is often part of a program known as systematic desensitisation [50]. For example, in the case of a woman with genital image concerns, she may be guided to first construct a hierarchy of fear or aversion. The hierarchy may include items such as looking at an image of a vulva in a book using, e.g., available resources [43–46], looking at a vulva in a video online, looking at her own vulva, inspecting her labia more closely with a hand-held mirror, asking a partner to look closely at her vulva and so on. These items are rank ordered on the hierarchy and the woman is exposed to the easiest item and progresses to the more challenging ones. After several weeks of consistent practice, she may be able to progress to the most distressing item (e.g., asking a partner to look closely at her vulva) with significantly less, or hopefully minimal, distress.

Another configuration of mirror exposure technique may involve the woman fixing her gaze on her reflection in the mirror, and describing her body from head to toe, and then from toe to head, using neutral descriptive language and avoiding judgement or value-laden words as if 'describing it to a blind person' [51]. Three sessions administered to women with significant body-related concerns were sufficient to significantly reduce body checking, body image avoidance, body dissatisfaction, depression and low self-esteem. Since this intervention combined exposure therapy (sustained looking at the feared object) together with mindful describing without judgement, the authors were not able to decipher which aspect of the treatment contributed to the positive outcomes. It seems that either modality, or their combination, would be suitable for women with concerns about vulvar image. More information about mindfulness-based approaches appears in the text that follows.

Cognitive Behaviour Therapy

Cognitive behavioural therapy (CBT) has been widely used in the treatment of body image distortions since the early 1980s. CBT rests on the premise that problematic thoughts which elicit negative emotions and behaviours have been learned and can be unlearned. Cognitive aspects included having participants challenge their own (typically distorted) perceptions of their body and replacing those with more accurate, balanced and compassionate thoughts. This approach entails teaching clients to observe how such negative thoughts make them feel (e.g., disgust, shame, fear, embarrassment) and act (e.g., avoid looking, looking obsessively, comparing to media images, etc.). By addressing the underlying unhelpful thoughts, clients can have a different emotional experience and behavioural outcome. CBT approaches to body image distortions have long been supported by the evidence [52] and, when compared to other stand-alone psychological treatments, have been shown to be highly effective [53]. Moreover, the benefits of CBT on body image persist even after therapy has ceased [54].

A Cochrane Review of the evidence finds CBT to be highly effective in the treatment of BDD [54]. However, we could not locate any specific study that directly evaluated CBT for the treatment of genital image concerns in women seeking FGCS. Nonetheless, given that this population of women experience cognitive, emotional and behavioural difficulties associated with their view of their vulvas [55] and the existing evidence for the efficacy of CBT for body image distortions more generally, a cognitive behavioural approach seems promising for women with genital image concerns.

Mindfulness-Based Approaches

Some of the behavioural exposure-based treatments for women with body image distortion involved having women describe out loud what they saw when they examined their body in a mirror. They were told, "Let your thoughts and emotions flow and do nothing to counter them" [56]. Such an approach decreased body dissatisfaction and emotional discomfort when women viewed their bodies. Although this approach was described as exposure therapy, and thus classified as a behaviour therapy intervention, the instruction of observing emotions and sensations without action falls in line with the broad array of mindfulness-based skills.

Mindfulness-based interventions evolved out of the work developed by Jon Kabat-Zinn and co-workers at University of Massachusetts Medical School from the late 1970s and tested originally in patients suffering from chronic and debilitating pains [57]. Mindfulness approaches involve moment-by-moment self-direction of attention to a particular target, such as the breath, body, sounds or thoughts. Sensations are observed compassionately and non-judgementally. An internet-based program of compassion training for undergraduate women with body image dissatisfaction included a compassionate body scan, an affectionate breathing exercise and a loving-kindness meditation focused on the body [58]. There were significant reductions in self-criticism and body image distress with the online treatment, but no changes in self-compassion itself. In the context of women experiencing genital self-image distortions, women may practise attending to physical and/or visual sensations of the vulva, and noticing those sensations moment-by-moment while letting go of the tendency to negatively label the area or the sensations.

Acceptance and commitment therapy (ACT) is considered a type of mindfulness-based intervention which rests heavily on the identification and clarification of the client's values. An unpublished doctoral dissertation by Anna Katherine Smith explored ACT as a treatment for women's genital and body dissatisfaction [59]. Smith developed a group intervention based on the principles of ACT that targeted genital self-image, sexual self-esteem, sexual openness and general body image. There were six 90-minute weekly sessions led by two experienced ACT facilitators and participants were college students with genital image concerns. The results of this excellent and comprehensive program are not yet available.

Sex Therapy

Approaches borrowed from sex therapy may be useful for the subgroup of women seeking FGCS who are particularly distressed about their sexual functioning, and/or believe that their partners are distressed about their sexuality and that FGCS will improve sexual satisfaction. Among the various sex therapy techniques utilised and studied over the past decades, sensate focus would be a suitable technique among this population. Sensate focus is a structured behavioural exercise developed by Masters and Johnson [60] and originally designed to address the widespread experience of anxiety that they observed in the men and women seeking sex therapy.

There are three stages to sensate focus: Stage 1 focuses on sequential touching of one partner and then the other, excluding the breasts and genitals, during which the giver of the touch was guided by his own curiosity, not by what he believed his partner liked. The recipient of the touch provided verbal feedback to the toucher about the qualities of the touch. After approximately 15 minutes, roles were reversed and the toucher now became the touchee. There was a focus on sensual, rather than erotic, pleasure, and overt sexual activity was often prohibited during the period of sensate focus practice. Stage 2 now included breast and genital touch and the goal remained to learn about the partner's body, rather than the overt creation of pleasure. Stage 3 involved mutual touching with the progressive reintroduction of intercourse. The therapist sought to monitor the couple's responses to prescribed homework activities, and would emphasise positive reinforcers while removing negative ones.

The outcomes of sensate focus have been studied systematically and Masters and Johnson found success rates in the range of 72–98% following sensate focus when it was practised daily, and only a 5% relapse rate after 5 years (1960). To this day, sensate focus remains a very popular technique [61] used for couples where there may be anxiety associated with sexual activity, perceptions of negative outcomes during a sexual encounter, significant distractions during sex or intense negative emotions associated with the encounter.

For women who are distressed about the look and feel of their genitals, sensate focus may offer them an opportunity to remain in the present moment while a partner touches the entire body, including the genitals. It may help the women to tune into positive sensual feelings while her eyes are closed, and it may enforce the role of relaxation while receiving touch, which gives way to subsequent sexual arousal. Though sensate focus has never been evaluated for addressing sexual or body image concerns among women seeking FGCS, our own clinical experience demonstrates its enormous utility. Future studies should seek to evaluate sensate focus in this population.

Although techniques drawn on behaviour therapy, CBT, mindfulness-based approaches and sex therapy can be useful in the treatment of women with genital image distress, the literature is scant on the evaluation of such approaches. We advocate strongly for researchers to evaluate their use of these strategies among women seeking FGCS.

Case Study 13.1 Leanne's Story

Leanne, a 24-year-old healthy young woman, was referred to her gynaecologist from her primary care provider after reporting increasing levels of anxiety and depression related to unhappiness with the size and shape of her labia. The gynaecologist carried out a clinical assessment and physical examination and concluded that Leanne was completely normal and that no labiaplasty would be offered. Leanne became extremely distressed. She agreed to be referred to a psychologist. The psychologist carried out a more extensive psychological and psychosexual assessment.

Leanne revealed that her reason for attending the appointment was to get the psychologist's approval for her to have surgery. She sought labiaplasty to reduce the asymmetry of her labia minora and to reduce the amount of protrusion. Leanne explained that for most of her life she had experienced discomfort from her labia "rubbing against one another" and that this had led to a need to "go to the bathroom five or six times per day to adjust myself". She noticed more discomfort during times of exercise and other outdoor activities, which she engages in avidly. On a scale of 0 to 10, Leanne rated the degree of her labial distress as 7 and said that her concerns had limited her physical activities such as running. She denied any vulval pain, and mainly expressed only discomfort.

When asked about her perception of normal vulval appearance, she revealed having consulted online media depicting women's genitals in the past year or so. The sources of those media tended to be pornography, which she reported that her boyfriend of the past 18 months had been viewing regularly. On occasions when they viewed pornography together, Leanne would fixate on

the small size of the actresses' labia and repeatedly ask her boyfriend if he preferred the vulvas of the actresses to her own. She would usually dismiss his reassurances.

Leanne's responses to a validated inventory suggested that she met criteria for BDD. On further probing, it was evident that she also felt dissatisfaction and discomfort about her body more generally. However, she felt that labiaplasty would improve her sexual function and mood, and the quality of her relationship. She worried about the impact of not having surgery, including her current partner leaving her.

In terms of mood, Leanne reported current symptoms of generalised as well as social anxiety and periodic episodes of depression throughout her teenage years. She reported one uncued panic attack several years ago. She described a moderate level of current stress that is likely attributable to balancing the demands of her university education, participation on a varsity athletic team, and involvement in her community as a volunteer. She reported trying to distract herself when she thought about her labia but found that it did not help. She appeared to understand the risks associated with labiaplasty. She has discussed this with a close friend of hers, who apparently encouraged Leanne to seek surgery.

Given Leanne's intrusive thoughts, and anxiety surrounding the fate of her current relationship, Leanne was encouraged to delay considering FGCS and instead focus her efforts on self-acceptance and address some of the biased and inaccurate beliefs she held about her body. The psychologist told her to consider putting surgery on hold, at least temporarily, and that if she still wished to pursue it in 3 months' time after completing a course of psychological therapy, the psychologist would explore this with her at that time. Leanne was diagnosed with Social Anxiety Disorder and BDD, and together with the psychologist, embarked on a 10-week program focusing on cognitive behavioural therapy as well as some components of mindfulness meditation. They agreed to meet weekly for an hour-long session.

In the initial stages of treatment, Leanne was taught to notice negative thoughts about her vulva when they happened. She tracked her mood, activity, and any precipitating events or thoughts prior to those irrational ones. With time, she discovered that she was more likely to have negative thoughts about her vulva when watching pornography, when changing in the locker room after sports, and in general when she was anxious or stressed about school. She was also taught to monitor her body sensations in response to those thoughts, and she found great relief in learning to practice progressive muscle relaxation. She learned that negative thoughts about her vulva triggered a series of physical reactions in her body, such as increased muscle tension, chest breathing, and light-headedness. She also learned, through CBT, that this constellation of body sensations led her to be even more vigilant about her body.

The psychologist also integrated into the treatment mindfulness meditation skills. Specifically, Leanne learned to view negative thoughts as passing mental events in the more spacious mind and that these events were neither factual nor needed to be followed up. She practised meditation to online instructions at least 15 minutes per day, and after approximately a month, she became more able to experience without reaction negative and judging thoughts as passing events. Over the course of our 2 months, Leanne's perceptions about her partner began to loosen, and she no longer believed that he would leave her.

By the end of 10 weeks, Leanne experienced a significant reduction in her anxiety associated with negative thoughts about her body. She was more able to de-escalate unhelpful thoughts when she noticed that they were beginning to arouse distressing emotions in her.

Conclusion

Women seeking FGCS may experience an array of psychological symptoms including anxiety, depression, poor body image and low self-esteem. Health care providers should be equipped to assess whether psychological symptoms are present, and evaluate the extent to which these are impacting the woman's desire for surgery. Whenever possible, we strongly advocate for the inclusion of a psychological assessment by an experienced practitioner, to adequately evaluate the psychological factors and work collaboratively with the physician. Where BDD may be contributing significantly to the body distortion and distress, we strongly recommend against pursuing FGCS and encourage the patient to acquire some psychological strategies to address the BDD first. There is a need for additional research on the long-term psychological outcomes of women seeking FGCS, whether they received surgery or not. Given the evidence of the benefits of psychological skills borrowed from behaviour therapy, cognitive behaviour therapy, mindfulness-based interventions, and sex therapy, we recommend that these approaches be utilised when working with women's genital image concerns, whether or not the women are currently seeking FGCS.

References

1. American Society of Plastic Surgeons. *Plastic surgery statistics teport.* 2016. Available from: www.plasticsurgery.org

2. Shridharani SM, Magarakis M, Manson PN, Rodriguez ED. Psychology of plastic and reconstructive surgery: A systematic clinical review. *Plast Reconstr Surg.* 2010;126(6):2243–51.

3. Manoloudakis N, Labiris G, Karakitsou N, Kim JB, Sheena Y, Niakas D. Characteristics of women who have had cosmetic breast implants that could be associated with increased suicide risk: A systematic review, proposing a suicide prevention model. *Arch Plast Surg.* 2015;42(2):131–42.

4. Moser SE, Aiken LS. Cognitive and emotional factors associated with elective breast augmentation among young women. *Psychol Health.* 2011;26(1):41–60.

5. Sharp G, Tiggemann M, Mattiske J. Factors that influence the decision to undergo labiaplasty: Media, relationships, and psychological well-being. *Aesthet Surg J.* 2016; 36: 469–78.

6. Braun V, Wilkinson S. Socio-cultural representations of the vagina. *J Reprod Infant Psychol.* 2001;19:17–32.

7. Bryce M, Brotto L, Todd N. Perceptions of female genitals by cis-women and their partners. *Under Review.*

8. Schick VR, Rima BN, Calabrese SK. Evulvalution: The portrayal of women's external genitalia and physique across time and the current Barbie doll ideals. *J Sex Res.* 2011;48: 74–81.

9. Bramwell R. Invisible labia: The representation of female external genitals in women's magazines. *Sex Relat Ther.* 2002;17:187–90.

10. Herbenick DL. The development and validation of a scale to measure attitudes toward women's genitals. *Int J Sex Health.* 2009;21:153–66.

11. Koning M, Zeijlmans IA, Bouman TK, van der Lei B. Female attitudes regarding labia minora appearance and reduction with consideration of media influence. *Aesthet. Surg J.* 2009;29: 65–71.

12. Jones B, Nurka C. Labiaplasty and pornography: A preliminary investigation. *Porn Stud.* 2015;2:62–75.

13. Herbenick D, Schick V, Reece M, et al. Pubic hair removal among women in the United States: Prevalence, methods, and characteristics. *J Sex Med.* 2010;7(10): 3322–30.

14. Moran C, Lee C. What's normal? Influencing women's perceptions of normal genitalia: An experiment

involving exposure to modified and nonmodified images. *BJOG.* 2014;121(6): 761–6.

15. Lloyd J, Crouch NS, Minto CL, Liao LM, Crieghton SM. Female genital appearance: 'Normality' unfolds. *BJOG.*2005;112(5): 643–6.

16. Green FJ. From clitoridectomies to 'designer vaginas': The medical construction of heteronormative female bodies and sexuality through female genital cutting. *Sex Evol Gend.*2005;7(2):153–87.

17. Liao LM, Creighton SM. Requests for cosmetic genitoplasty: How should healthcare providers respond? *BMJ.* 2007;334(7603): 1090–2.

18. Godlee F. Promoting cosmetic surgery. *BMJ.* 2012;345: e7535.

19. Liao LM, Taghinejadi N, Creighton SM. An analysis of the content and clinical implications of online advertisements for female genital cosmetic surgery. *BMJ Open.* 2012;2: e001908. doi:10.1136/bmjopen-2012-001908.

20. Barbara G, Facchin F, Meschia M, Vercellini P. 'The first cut is the deepest': A psychological, sexological and gynecological perspective on female genital cosmetic surgery. *Acta Obstet Gynecol Scand.* 2015;94 (9): 915–20.

21. Bramwell R, Morland C. Genital appearance satisfaction in women: The development of a questionnaire and exploration of correlates. *J Reprod Infant Psychol.* 2009;27(1):15–27.

22. Rouzier R, Louis-Sylvestre C, Paniel BJ, Haddad B. Hypertrophy of labia minora: Experience with 163 reductions. *Am J Obstet Gynecol.* 2000;182(1):35–40.

23. Veale D, Eshkevari E, Ellison N, et al. Psychological characteristics and motivation of women seeking labiaplasty. *Psychol Med.* 2014;44(3):555–66.

24. Mitchell KR, Mercer CH, Ploubidis GB, et al. Sexual function in Britain: Findings from the third National Survey of Sexual Attitudes and Lifestyles (Natsal-3). *Lancet* 2013;382(9907):1817–29.

25. Brotto L, Atallah S, Johnson-Agbakwu C, et al. Psychological and interpersonal dimensions of sexual function and dysfunction. *J Sex Med.* 2016;13(4):538–71.

26. Goodman MP, Placik OJ, Benson III RH, et al. A large multicenter outcome study of female genital plastic surgery. *J Sex Med.* 2010;7(4 Pt1):1565–77.

27. Goodman M, Fashler S, Miklos JR, Moore RD, Brotto LA. The sexual, psychological, and body image health of women undergoing elective vulvovaginal plastic/cosmetic procedures: a pilot study. *Am J Cosmetic Surg.* 2011;28(4): 219–26.

28. O'sullivan LF, Brotto LA, Byers ES, Majerovich JA, Wuest JA. Prevalence and characteristics of sexual functioning among sexually experienced middle to late adolescents. *J Sex Med.* 2014;11(3):630–41.

29. Sorice SC, Li AY, Canales FL, Furnas HJ. Why women request Labiaplasty. *Plast Reconstr Surg.* 2017;139 (4):856–63.

30. Sharp G, Tiggemann M, Mattiske J. Predictors of consideration of labiaplasty: An extension of the tripartite influence model of beauty ideals. *Psych Women Q.* 2015;39(2):182–93.

31. Veale D, Eshkevari E, Ellison N. Cardozo L, Robinson D, Kavouni A. Validation of genital appearance satisfaction scale and the cosmetic procedure screening scale for women seeking labiaplasty. *J Psychosom Obstet Gynecol.* 2013;34(1):46–52.

32. Lee K, Guy A, Dale J, Wolke D. Adolescent desire for cosmetic surgery: Associations with bullying and psychological functioning. *Plast Reconstr Surg.* 2017;139(5): 1109–18.

33. American Psychiatric Association. *Diagnostic and statistical manual of mental disorders (DSM-5®).* Washington, DC: American Psychiatric Publishing; 2013.

34. Veale D, Bewley A. Body dysmorphic disorder. *BMJ.* 2015;350: h2278.

35. Fang A, Wilhelm S. Clinical features, cognitive biases, and treatment of body dysmorphic disorder. *Annu Rev Clin Psychol.* 2015;11:187–212.

36. Liao LM, Michala L, Creighton SM. Labial surgery for well women: A review of the literature. *BJOG.* 2010;117 (1):20–5.

37. Shaw D, Lefebvre G, Bouchard C, et al. Female genital cosmetic surgery. *J Obstet Gynaecol Can.* 2013;35 (12):1108–12.

38. Sharp G, Mattiske J, Vale KI. Motivations, expectations, and experiences of labiaplasty: A qualitative study. *Aesthet Surg J.* 2016;36(8):920–8.

39. Royal College of Obstetricians and Gynaecologists. Ethical considerations in relation to female genital cosmetic surgery (FGCS). 2013.

40. Lykkebo AW, Drue HC, Lam JUH, Guldberg R. The size of labia minora and perception of genital appearance: A cross-sectional study. *J Low Genit Tract Dis.* 2017;21(3):198–203.

41. Sharp G, Tiggemann M. Educating women about normal female genital appearance variation. *Body Image.* 2016;16:70–8.

42. Laan E, Martoredjo DK, Hesselink S, Snijders N, van Lunsen RHW. Young women's genital self-image and effects of exposure to pictures of natural vulvas. *J Psychosom Obstet Gynecol.* 2017;38(4):249–55.

43. Karras N. *Petals.* Heath, TX: Crystal River Publishing; 2003.

127

44. Women's Health Victoria. Labia Library. Available from: www.labialibrary.org.au/

45. McCartney J. Great Wall of Vagina. Fine Art Studios. Available from: www.greatwallofvagina.co.uk/home.

46. Drysdale K, Russell A. Labiaplasty. *Hungry Beast: ABC1*, 12 April 2010, https://vimeo.com/180883108.

47. Honigman RJ, Phillips KA, Castle DJ. A review of psychosocial outcomes for patients seeking cosmetic surgery. *Plast Reconstr Surg.* 2004;113(4):1229–37.

48. Brohede S, Wingren G, Wijma B, Wijma K. Validation of the Body Dysmorphic Disorder Questionnaire in a community sample of Swedish women. *Psychiatry Res.* 2013;210:647–52.

49. Phillips KA, Hollander E, Rasmussen SA, Aronowitz BR, DeCaria C, Goodman WK. A severity rating scale for body dysmorphic disorder: Development, reliability, and validity of a modified version of the Yale–Brown Obsessive Compulsive Scale. *Psychopharmacol Bull.* 1997;33:17–22.

50. McCallie MS, Blum CM, Hood CJ. Progressive muscle relaxation. *J Human Behav Soc Environ.* 2006;13:51–66.

51. Delinsky SS, Wilson GT. Mirror exposure for the treatment of body image disturbance. *Int J Eating Dis.* 2006;39:108–16.

52. Rosen JC, Cado S, Silberg NT, Srebnik D, Wendt S. Cognitive behavior therapy with and without size perception training for women with body image disturbance. *Behav Ther.* 1990;21:481–98.

53. Jarry JL, Berardi K. Characteristics and effectiveness of stand-alone body image treatments: A review of the empirical literature. *Body Image.* 2004;1:319–33.

54. Ipser JC, Sander C, Stein DJ. Pharmacotherapy and psychotherapy for body dysmorphic disorder. *Cochrane Database Syst Rev.* 2009;1:CD005332.

55. Veale D, Naismith I, Eshkevari E, et al. Psychosexual outcome after labiaplasty: A prospective case-comparison study. *Int Urogyn J.* 2014;25(6):831–9.

56. Diaz-Ferrer S, Rodriguez-Ruiz S, Ortega-Roldan B, Mata-Martin JL, Fernandez-Santaella CF. Psychophysiological changes during pure vs guided mirror exposure therapies in women with high body dissatisfaction: What are they learning about their bodies? *Eur Eating Dis Rev.* 2017;25:562–9.

57. Kabat-Zinn J. An outpatient program in behavioral medicine for chronic pain patients based on the practice of mindfulness meditation: Theoretical considerations and preliminary results. *Gen Hosp Psychiatry.* 1982;4(1):33–47.

58. Toole AM, Craighead LW. Brief self-compassion meditation training for body image distress in young adult women. *Body Image.* 2016;19:104112.

59. Smith AK. *Female genital image self-consciousness: Using acceptance and commitment therapy in a group setting with college-aged women.* Unpublished doctoral dissertation. (Order No. 10285929). Available from ProQuest Dissertations & Theses Global (1914912987): http://ezproxy.library.ubc.ca/login?url=https://search.proquest.com/docview/1914912987?accountid=14656

60. Masters WH, Johnson VE. *Human sexual inadequacy.* Boston: Little, Brown & Co.; 1970.

61. Weiner L, Avery-Clark C. Sensate focus: Clarifying the Masters and Johnson's model. *Sex Relat Ther.* 2014;29 (3):307–19.

Addressing Female Genital Dissatisfaction and Distress
The Role of Nurses and Midwives

Yana Richens and Louise Williams

Introduction

"Do I look normal down there?" This is a question asked by women that many nurses and midwives are all too familiar with. Nurses who work in cervical screening, sexual health and specialist gynaecology clinics have ample opportunities to assist women and girls to explore their genital appearance concerns, to offer reassurances, to signpost to women-centred resources and to offer appropriate advice and triaging. This is also true of the midwives for whom genital examination of women is routine.

In this chapter, we begin by critiquing nursing and midwifery training for not adequately addressing female body distress in general, not least because the professions are themselves staffed mainly by women who are subjected to the same social pressures as the female patients. We will provide a range of clinical scenarios whereby nurses and midwives can offer women useful input. Although we make references to 'women' and 'girls' in this chapter, we acknowledge that not all people with female-typical genitals identify as such.

Limitations of Nursing and Midwifery Education

In recent years, there has been a shift in nursing and midwifery education away from hospital-based clinical training to an academic degree–based model in the UK [1]. According to UK's Nursing and Midwifery Council standards for pre-registration nursing education, all nurses and midwives must possess a broad knowledge of the structure and functions of the human body [2]. However, there is significant variability in how this broad brief is translated by training programmes that are governed by the Higher Education Institutes (HEI). Research shows that practitioners lack confidence in explaining the bio-scientific

rationale for their clinical practice [1]. When it comes to gynaecology, the coverage is generally thin and invariably limited to reproductive physiology, with very little information on genital anatomy. For midwives, the female anatomy is covered in greater detail, but not to the extent that they can confidently address women's concerns about genital appearance and function.

Nurses and midwives have fought long and hard for the professional autonomy that they currently enjoy. In many countries, practitioners are granted prescribing rights. In the UK nurse prescribing is well established, with more than 54,000 nurse and midwife prescribers in 2012 [3]. Many more independently offer specialist clinics in acute and community hospitals. They provide independent services in sexual health, family planning, birth injury, female genital mutilation and paediatric and adolescent gynaecology, to name a few. The pressure to acquire bio-scientific knowledge for effective professional practice has increased. However, in all of these specialties, there are implicit and explicit requirements for nursing and midwifery professionals to offer patient-centred or whole-person care [4]. As such, they need to be skilled at detecting emotional concerns. It is important for professional training decision makers to ensure that a balance between bio-scientific education and consultation training is achieved in nursing and midwifery training.

Currently, there are 285,893 nurses and health visitors and 21,596 midwives (whole-time equivalent) registered in the UK [5], of whom 89% are female and 11% are male [6]. Women working in these professions are subjected to the same social pressures on gendered appearances, functions and roles as the women for whom they provide care. A thorough education on female genital anatomy and functions should be seen as much as training for the professional as it is a health education intervention for the woman.

While we discuss how nurses and midwives can assist other women, we must also reflect on how social pressures on female appearances may have shaped our own personal preferences and responses to patient and client concerns. If women in the general population are getting their information from the media, in what way are female nurses and midwives different? If we fail to question ourselves, our ignorance will continue to remain in the blind spot, and unhelpful and unprofessional anecdotes pertaining to women seeking information and reassurance being told to have their genitals 'tidied up' will surface time and again. The opportunity for empathic reflections and reassurances is repeatedly lost.

A Life Course Understanding of Female Genital Anatomy

Girls and women at any age can feel deeply distressed about their genitals, regardless of how they may appear. The reasons for seeking surgery are variable. Some feel that aspects of their lifestyle are restricted by the inner labia protruding beyond the outer labia (e.g., they find wearing tight clothes and swimsuits uncomfortable or embarrassing). However, research shows that there are no differences in labial dimensions between women who seek labiaplasty and those who do not [7]. Very few men are known to have their genital mass surgically reduced in order to feel more comfortable riding a bicycle or a horse. Therefore female genital distress is gendered. Psychologists have pointed out that even small sensations in a body part can be experienced as intolerable due to their emotional valence.

Throughout the lifespan, the female genitalia change considerably in size, shape and colouration. Our collective failure to recognise and value diversity in body and sexuality is a blessing to the FGCS industry, which in turn keeps us in ignorance. As we present a life course understanding for nurses and midwives in this section, we offer case vignettes to demonstrate good practice.

Puberty

Prepubertal girls generally have smaller inner labia which are often not visible without close inspection. In response to pubertal hormonal changes, the inner labia and the clitoris become much more noticeable. This is entirely normal. During this developmental process, one side can start growing first and both sides usually even out after a while. However, perfect symmetry does not always ensue. This too is normal. The lack of education on vulval structure and appearance diversity combined with popular but biased representations can leave some girls and often their mothers feeling unsure.

Case Study 14.1

A Teenage Girl Seeks Labiaplasty with Parental Support

Hannah is 16 years old. Accompanied by her mother, Hannah meets with her general practitioner (GP) to ask if she can have her inner labia made smaller. In the electronic notes "normal" and "floods of tears" are mentioned. The GP is non-committal and makes an appointment for Hannah and her mother to meet with the practice nurse. Accompanied by her mother, Hannah comes for her appointment. She looks embarrassed and signals to her mother to begin the conversation with the nurse. Her mother says: "I'm worried about my daughter. She gets really upset about how she looks down below … She showed me it. It [the inner labia] doesn't look right. I don't remember that. She wants to have the surgery and I think that will really help." The nurse verifies this with Hannah, who continues the conversation by stating quietly but vehemently how much she hates the way her inner labia look and feel. When asked how she would like her vulva to look, Hannah states

---

BOX 14.1 Example Responses and Comments

Responses	*Comments*
"The doctor thinks you're normal, Hannah. It's how you feel though, I understand that. I see lots of girls with poor body image these days. But surgery is not always the answer. I'm happy to talk to you about why you are absolutely normal. What do you think, mum? Or is Hannah not better off seeing our counsellor?"	The content of the message is not wrong. However, the empathy is hollow. It dismisses the young person's very real concerns, making it difficult for her to work with you.
"Wait a while and see how you feel. I understand surgery is a day case. It is available privately if you can't get it for free. Obviously if you continue to be bothered by this and you think it can really help you, then no one can stop you."	Here, before any alternative views are explored, the nurse normalises surgery which is invasive and irrevocable but does not address any biomedical concerns.

BOX 14.2 Outline of a More Helpful Consultation

Steps	*Additional Notes*
Welcome both and praise the mother for being supportive of her daughter. Always inform young people of their right to privacy and confidentiality. Check with Hannah if she would like her mother to stay in the room. If so, mention that you might still ask her mother to leave the room for part of the consultation if Hannah were willing. This will provide you time to provide a confidential space where the young person can disclose any sensitive information which may embarrass them in front of their parents, such as having been sexually active. Try and build rapport with the daughter and the mother. Manage expectations by asking what they have in mind by way of an outcome of the consultation. If support for surgery is mentioned, discuss that this may not ensue but that you are committed to helping them explore a range of options.	The nurse should demonstrate her recognition of the sensitivity of the situation and reassure Hannah and her mother, both vulnerable to shame, that their feelings are valid and they are right to seek help. The nurse's professionalism will help to gain Hannah and her mother's confidence and trust.
Invite Hannah to tell you about her concerns in her own words, e.g., "Tell me about your worries … " If Hannah is willing, encourage her to elaborate, e.g., "Can you say a bit more … ?". Acknowledge that her feelings are real, e.g., "Your distress is real. There's no right or wrong in our feelings. Many girls tell me they feel unhappy about their body. Before we discuss how to approach your concerns, it's important we talk more." Ask Hannah about her life in general – to place the problem in context and to get to know Hannah better.	The health concerns of the young person and her parent should be properly acknowledged. Note whether the young person appears to be withdrawn or anxious and explore current coping strategies which may be positive (e.g., talk to friends about her feelings) or negative (e.g., self-harm/alcohol misuse). As well as that, explore any family (e.g., parents not getting on) and peer problems (e.g., bullying).
Ask Hannah what kind of information she has used, e.g., has she viewed the web pages of cosmetic surgery companies and their 'before-and-after' picture galleries? This could be a talking point before looking at resources which show a range of genital diversity.	An internet survey suggests that 16- to 24-year-olds are more likely to seek health information and advice online than from health professionals [8].
Seek permission before offering Hannah and her mother some images on vulval appearance diversity such as the Labia Library [9], e.g., "Would it be ok if we look together at some images of 'normal'? And then you can tell me what you think."	Recent studies have shown that many adult women have limited knowledge of the different parts of the vulva, their function and genital diversity [10].
Make a further appointment for a follow-up discussion.	

that her inner labia should not be showing and that by "leaking" out of the outer labia, they rub together and cause soreness. Hannah's mother further adds that Hannah has always been a healthy and happy child without any emotional problems. She says Hannah is not vain and is never bothered about how she looks, but that it is "not right" that her labia are "hanging down." Both daughter and mother want to emphasise that they are not considering surgery "at a whim" and that Hannah has been unhappy about her labia for several years. In Boxes 14.1 and 14.2, we explore potential ways of approaching the conversation with mother and daughter.

Notes on Educational Intervention

As you acknowledge feelings using the patient's own words, you can also reframe denigrating wording by offering positive or neutral vocabularies (e.g., 'sensitive tissue' instead of 'extra skin'). You can do this implicitly or explicitly: "Psychologists tell us that the way we talk to ourselves can affect how we feel. I would like to suggest that we try to avoid words that make a situation seem worse than it actually is." Furthermore, always use correct terms for the different parts of the genitalia and never refer to the vulva as the vagina. For example: "This is the clitoris. It's made up of the glans which is usually hidden by the clitoral hood. The glans is very sensitive so the hood keeps it protected from rubbing. The glans gets a bit bigger during sexual arousal because of the extra blood flow. The only function of the clitoris is sexual pleasure."

Here is another example of how to communicate to patients: "You've got two sets of labia, the inside and the outside ones. The so called inner labia, despite its name, is visible for most women and, for some women, one side more so than the other. They usually look a little wrinkly after puberty and sometimes even before, because they are soft and stretchy. They have an important job to do – to protect your vaginal opening and experts say nowadays they contribute to sexual pleasure."

As a third example of how to give information: "It is normal for the outer labia (lips) to grow bigger and for the clitoris to become more prominent. What a shame no one talks about these normal changes during puberty and later, causing so many girls and even older women to worry."

Notes on Genital Examination

Hannah should not be examined again unless you are especially confident and skilled in performing genital examinations [11]. The most likely outcome of another examination is that you will, like Hannah's GP, see a normal vulva. However, it may be an opportunity for Hannah to pinpoint the exact area that she is worried about. You can also teach Hannah about the different parts of the vulva on an examination couch using a mirror so she can see her own genitals. Alternatively, you can use images from online resources such as the Labia Library [8]. It is best practice to ask Hannah how she would like to do this.

The examination must be discussed first and consent obtained, including whether the mother is to be present. A chaperone should also be available. Ensure that enough time is allocated and that you are not disturbed halfway through. Have all materials at hand (e.g., lubrication and swabs if needed).

Notes on Clinical Advice Following an Examination

If there is visible abnormal discharge or the young person is sexually active, you may need to take swabs in order to rule out vaginal infections. During the visual inspection it is important to check the vulval skin for any sores/patches of discolouration which may indicate a dermatological complaint requiring further investigation. Accurate records during and following the consultation are essential.

Younger women often complain that their labia are painful and get in the way or are prone to recurrent infections. This can be related to lifestyle practices, such as pubic hair removal. Girls and women should be informed about the sensitivity of their labial skin and the damage that shaving and waxing can do to the area. An alternative is to trim the hair rather than removing it

entirely. Soap and wipes including those specified as 'suitable for intimate use' are best avoided, as are shaving gels and vaginal deodorants. A discussion around the natural, normal smell of the vagina should take place. At menarche girls are more likely to initially use sanitary towels during menstruation; this can cause chaffing. Additionally, tight-fitting 'thong' style underwear can lead to genital soreness. It can be helpful to draw attention to the effects of some of these lifestyle practices.

Pubic hair grooming has become increasingly prevalent in the twenty-first century. In 2016 a study reported that out of 3,316 American women surveyed, 2,778 (84%) reported a history of lifetime pubic hair grooming [12]. A total of 875 (31.5% women) reported grooming because they believe it makes their genitals more attractive, and 586 (21.1%) reported grooming because of partner preference. When asked about situations for which they groom, women reported sex as the most common reason (1,544 [55.6%]) and health care professional visit (1,111 [40.0%]). Factors associated with pubic grooming include being younger, unmarried and increased sexual activity. It is advisable for women during pregnancy to refrain from shaving due to increased possibility of cutting themselves as the pubis becomes less visible. Women need reassurance regarding the physical changes to their body during pregnancy and further reassurance about what will happen during labour.

Pregnancy

The vagina is transformed during puberty and pregnancy and after menopause. Some pregnant and postpartum women can become confused and worried about changes for which they are ill prepared. Through professional education, clinical experience and effective supervision, nurses and midwives should confidently explore women's concerns and tailor their information and guidance. They should be familiar with the vast resources that have been developed but underutilised and learn how to use them effectively (see Resources in the appendix).

When a woman first becomes pregnant she may notice some changes in her vagina in appearance and smell. These physical signs are more noticeable in women who remove pubic hair. Blood flow to the vagina is increased, making the vaginal tissue softer. It is a feeling of "heaviness" due to the increased blood flow. Historically it was the lilac discolouration of the vagina and cervix, called Jacquemier's sign after a French obstetrician (1806–1879), which led to confirmation of the pregnancy (although this is also symptomatic of pelvic tumours, such as fibroids). The increased blood flow results in pulsating of the uterine arteries, and can be felt on vaginal examination in the lateral fornices (referred to as Osiander's sign). The increase in venous engorgement results in the presence of an increased vaginal discharge which is white and has a reduced pH (alkaline) due to the presence of raised oestrogen level. Although these signs are no longer used to confirm a pregnancy, women attending antenatal clinics for their first booking appointment often bring up the issue of increased discharge and changes in the shape and feeling of her vagina. However, this should not be discounted as normal. Always take time to listen to the woman's concerns, before discounting it as a normal aspect of pregnancy. It is also interesting to consider what may have changed. In the author's experience as a midwife [YR] such issues were not discussed so openly 30 years ago. This leads us to ask the question of what, if anything, has changed regarding pregnancy.

Case Study 14.2

A Woman Seeks 'Vaginal Tightening'

Claudia is a 31-year-old woman who has a follow-up appointment with the community midwife six weeks after the birth of her first baby. When the examination is completed, Claudia is quiet, with her eyes cast down. She hesitates and then asks the midwife how "it" looks "down below." What Claudia wants to know is whether to the midwife, her vagina is too open, as a friend has said something about 'vaginal laxity' after childbirth. Claudia wants to know if the introitus of her vagina is too visible and if so, whether this is the result of having had a big baby. Claudia would also like to know what the current opinions are on vaginal tightening after childbirth, and whether it "works"? In Boxes 14.3 and 14.4, we offer steps for having a helpful conversation with Claudia.

Notes on Educational Intervention

As you acknowledge feelings using the patient's own words, you can also role model questioning some of the denigrating concepts. For example, what is 'vaginal laxity'? If a vagina is too loose, it is too loose for what? It is also important to reassure women that they can derive sexual satisfaction in a multitude of ways,

and that how people think about sex can profoundly shape experience. There are many useful tools for discussing female sexuality with patients and clients, such as the New View campaign and the Sexualisation Report [13] available on the internet.

Notes on Birth Injuries

In a recent qualitative study [14], some women reported a fear of perineal tearing and potential physical trauma from childbirth. Fear of damage to the pelvic floor is often cited as a primary reason for requesting a Caesarean section by women with a low-risk pregnancy [15]. When women sustain a tear from a vaginal delivery, it is important to help them make an informed choice as to whether or not to be sutured.

A Cochrane Review looked at surgical repair versus non-surgical repair of perineal tears [16]. The review included two randomised controlled trials involving 154 women. The review focused on perineal pain and healing and did not include body image. The author's [YR] experience of running a birth injury clinic for

---

BOX 14.3 Example Responses and Comments

Responses	Comments
"If it were me I wouldn't bother. I'm not sure if it works anyway."	Claudia may have thought long and hard before raising such a sensitive topic. This may even be the real reason for the appointment. Such a casual comment is likely to be disappointing and undermining. In any case the midwife should not influence the patient by stating her personal choice.
"I'm afraid I know nothing about it. I've never come across it. You need to be careful about these ads you know. You don't want to make things worse for yourself."	This can make Claudia feel like she is the only person with such a worry when she may well be expressing something that many women have either fleeting worries or serious concerns about.
"That makes sense if you're worried about it. At the end of the day it's your choice what to do with your body isn't it? People have all sorts of things done."	This flash and ill-considered response almost reinforces the idea that it is right that women should do "all sorts of things" to themselves to cope with their body insecurities.

BOX 14.4 Outline of a Helpful Consultation

Steps	*Additional Notes*
Reassure Claudia that you want to listen to her concerns. Manage expectations by asking what she would like the outcome of the conversation to be. If your opinion is sought, discuss that this may not be possible but that you can support her to clarify her concerns.	The midwife should demonstrate her recognition of the sensitivity of the situation and reassure the patient who is vulnerable to shame and embarrassment. The midwife's professionalism will provide relief for a problem that may have been preoccupying Claudia for some time.
Invite Claudia to elaborate on her concerns. Acknowledge her feelings. Inquire about life in general – to place the problem in context and to get to know her better.	Explore the context (e.g., feeling insecure about a current relationship) or specific incidents (e.g., teased by a previous partner). Note whether Claudia appears withdrawn or anxious and inquire how she is coping as a first-time mum.
Ask where her perception of vaginal laxity comes from and how she may have heard of 'vaginal rejuvenation' (e.g., from a sexual partner, media, web pages of cosmetic surgery companies). Explain that some procedures are not formally recognisable and are without an evidence base.	It is possible that women have not considered such denigrating ideas about their vagina until they see an advertisement for 'vaginal rejuvenation.' Alternatively Claudia and her partner may be concerned about their sex life after a baby.
Validate Claudia's distress but also mention that many myths about sex can make women and men feel insecure. Invite her to look at some sexual health information together and discuss how she feels. Offer to see her again for a follow-up. This is also an opportunity to provide information on pelvic floor exercises.	This may be a useful point to debunk the myth about 'tightness' in genital intercourse as the path to satisfying sexual intimacy. If there are relationship or sexual problems they are likely to be complex, so that triaging to expert services may need to be considered.

postnatal women found that quite often women who attend clinic are not satisfied when a perineal/labial tear has been left to heal unsutured. The general consensus is that they were not informed of the pros and cons of not having 'stiches'. Not suturing can result in the labia minora not being symmetrical, and in some cases a very clear split in the labia minora can be identified. This can leave some women feeling embarrassed and upset. They may voice concerns about their future sex life. This is not helped by flippant remarks of male partners such as," Just put an extra couple of stitches in while you are there." While comments are often said to lighten the situations, some women say they remember them for the rest of their lives.

Although the majority of women feel that surgical repair is the only option, the Cochrane review concludes, "Until further evidence becomes available, clinicians' decisions whether to suture or not can be based on their clinical judgement and the women's preference after informing them about the lack of long-term outcomes and the possible chance of a slower wound healing process" [16]. However, the author would suggest that following birth, if the woman has sustained a vaginal or labial tear, then discussion with the woman should also include the possible appearance of the perineum/labia if left unsutured. This would enable the woman to make a fully informed decision.

Menopause

Menopause is a normal biological transition in mid-life or many women, as they reach the end of reproductive life and stop menstruating. Usually it is defined by the absence of menses for 12 consecutive months in the absence of any pathology [17]. As a result of the decreasing oestrogen levels, a significant proportion of women experience vasomotor symptoms (sweats and flushes) and musculoskeletal symptoms (joint and muscle pain); some women report a lowering of mood for a while or some fluctuations. In addition, the drop in oestrogen exposure can cause thinning and shrinking of the tissues of the vulva, vagina, urethra and bladder. This could lead to symptoms such as vaginal dryness, vaginal irritation, a frequent need to urinate, urinary tract infections and painful intercourse.

An online survey by the British Menopause Society in 2017 highlighted that the menopause can result in life-changing events for both women and their partners [18]. Three-quarters of women who took part in the survey stated that menopause caused them to change their life and more than half said it had a negative impact on their lives. Fifty-one per cent of women stated that the menopause affected their sex life and 38% of partners reported feeling helpless when it came to supporting their partners during menopause.

Case Study 14.3

A Middle-Aged Woman Opportunistically Seeks Reassurance

Suri is a 48-year-old woman who has met a male partner after her divorce and comes for a sexual health check. The nurse needs to do a speculum examination in order to collect samples. As she is about to insert the speculum Suri says to the nurse "I'm so, so sorry that you have to do this. I don't know how you do your job. Is my vagina normal? It feels a bit different these days." In Boxes 14.5 and 14.6, we discuss potential ways of thinking with Suri about her concerns.

Sexual health nurses should be knowledgeable about the physical and potential psychosocial changes associated with menopause without falling into the trap of medicalising what is a normal transition for the vast majority of women. In conversation with women it is important to avoid reinscribing the sexism in the wider culture that overvalues youthfulness and devalues ageing in females. It is worth bearing in mind that in cultures where menopause is not framed by a negative narrative and/or where women's social status is elevated after menopause, women report far fewer physical symptoms and psychological difficulties compared to Western women. However, even in Westernised societies, many women report that cessation of menses and freedom from pregnancy bring relief. Many women welcome the chance to focus on their own health and well-being for the first time in adulthood. Many return to full-time gainful employment; others resume their education.

The National Institute for Health and Care Excellence (NICE) guideline on menopause provides current and comprehensive advice on conservative management [17]. By de-pathologising ageing and the signs of ageing, nurses have the potential to help women to make the most of the second half of their adult life. Freedom from unbearable social pressures to meet exacting standards of conventional female beauty could be an empowering message for mid-aged women, and nurses have ample opportunities to facilitate it.

The Future

In the British Society for Paediatric and Adolescent Gynaecology's position statement on labiaplasty [11], frontline and specialist clinicians are encouraged to improve their skills and confidence in educating and supporting girls with genital appearance concerns and their families. This message is equally relevant for midwives and nurses who provide care for women across the lifespan.

Midwives and nurses are more likely to be female. They work in clinical areas where they come into regular contact with female patients and many regularly examine women. Together they have more opportunities than any other health professional to talk to girls and women about their genital concerns and offer quality education and advice. Their potential contribution to develop non-surgical alternatives to address female genital concerns is vast. Thus far though, this opportunity is generally missed.

We hope that this chapter demonstrates the useful work that midwives and nurses could do if they were to take more interest in the growing dissatisfaction and distress that underpins FGCS and work with experts in other disciplines to stamp out its unhealthy rise. To make the most of their professional careers, there may have to be some changes in the training curricula of nurses and midwives. Fundamentally, a better balance in focus needs to be struck between knowledge of the biosciences and skills in interaction with patients and organisations. Furthermore, midwifery and nursing training programmes should encourage female students and trainees to openly explore their own experiences of the unbearable pressures to manage their bodies to satisfy the shifting cultural ideals.

BOX 14.5 Example Responses and Comments	
Responses	*Comments*
"Oh, now that you mention it, I can see that your labia are hanging down quite a bit. Have you spoken to anyone about this before?"	This response may well confirm Suri's worst fear when she is only casually seeking reassurances that she has nothing to worry about.
"Yes you do feel a little dry and tense down here. Is this normal for you?"	The use of "down there" may be experienced as condoning shame and embarrassment. In most situations it is preferable to model openness and check that Suri knows about the different parts of the vulva and their function.

BOX 14.6 Outline of a More Helpful Consultation

Steps	*Additional Notes*
Welcome Suri and congratulate her on her new relationship.	The nurse should recognise that the change in relationship is a big step for Suri. Demonstrating a real interest in her new relationship will help to gain Suri's confidence and trust.
Take the opportunity to ask Suri when her last period was and her knowledge and understanding of menopause.	Unless you notice anything unusual, reassure Suri that her vulva looks healthy.
Clarify with Suri her concerns and offer the opportunity to explore them with her during or after the consultation.	Use the opportunity to discuss sexual health with Suri and the possibility of vaginal dryness which may result in uncomfortable intercourse or a loss of interest in sex. It is also important to draw attention to the fact that the risk of sexually transmitted diseases remains even after menopause.
Provide time and space for Suri to discuss with you any concerns both physical and psychological and encourage her to elaborate. Acknowledge that her feelings are real. Ask about her life in general – to place the problem in context and to get to know Suri better.	This is a good opportunity to discuss any concerns such as feelings about becoming older and/or sons and daughters leaving home.
If appropriate, and a rapport between nurse and patient is sensed, ask permission to open up the opportunity for education, e.g., "Now that I have your attention, if you're not in a hurry, would you like me to show you some materials that are available to the public about what's normal for female genitalia?"	Use the resources that you feel most comfortable with using (see Resources in the appendix) that emphasise the spectrum of normality. This may open the discussion on the natural and normal changes associated with menopause.

Acknowledgements

Both authors thank Lih-Mei Liao for her generous input and guidance, and Sarah Creighton for her suggestions and encouragement. YR further thanks University College London Centre for Nursing and Midwifery Research for granting academic time to complete this work.

References

1. Taylor V, Ashelford S, Fell P, Goacher P. Biosciences in nurse education: Is the curriculum fit for practice? Lecturers' views and recommendations from across the UK. *J Clin Nurs*. 2015;24(19–20):2797–2806.

2. Standards for pre-registration nursing education. Nmc.org.uk. 2017. Available from: www.nmc.org.uk/standards/additional-standards/standards-for-pre-registration-nursing-education/

3. RCN Fact Sheet Nurse Prescribing in the UK. My.rcn.org.uk. 2017. Available from: https://my.rcn.org.uk/__data/assets/pdf_file/0008/443627/Nurse_Prescribing_in_the_UK_-_RCN_Factsheet.pdf

4. Nursing and Midwifery Council. Nursing and Midwifery Council Standards for Competence for Registered Nurses, 2014. www.nmc.org.uk/standards/additional-standards/standards-for-competence-for-registered-nurses/

5. NHS statistics, facts and figures. Nhsconfed.org. 2017. Available from: www.nhsconfed.org/resources/key-statistics-on-the-nhs

6. Annual Equality and Diversity Report. Nmc.org.uk. 2016. Available from: www.nmc.org.uk/globalassets/sitedocuments/annual_reports_and_accounts/equality-and-diversity-report-2015–16.pdf

7. Crouch N, Deans R, Michala L, Liao L, Creighton S. Clinical characteristics of well women seeking labial reduction surgery: A prospective study. *BJOG*. 2011;118(12):1507–10.

8. An app a day keeps the doctor away: 16–24s more likely to trust websites for health advice than professionals. Mintel.com. 2018. Available from: www.mintel.com/press-centre/social-and-lifestyle/an-app-a-day-keeps-the-doctor-away-16-24s-more-likely-to-trust-websites-for-health-advice-than-professionals

9. Home.. Labialibrary.org.au. 2018. Available from: www.labialibrary.org.au/

10. McDougall L. Towards a clean slit: how medicine and notions of normality are shaping female genital aesthetics. *Cult Health Sex*. 2013;15(7):774–87.

11. Position Statement: Labial reduction surgery (labiaplasty) on adolescents. Britspag.org. 2013. Available from: www.britspag.org/sites/default/files/

downloads/Labiaplasty%20%20final%20Position%20S
tatement.pdf

12. Rowen T, Gaither T, Awad M, Osterberg E, Shindel A, Breyer B. Pubic hair grooming prevalence and motivation among women in the United States. *JAMA Dermatol*. 2016;152(10):1106.

13. The sexualization report.Thesexualizationreport.files. wordpress.com. 2013. Available from: https://thesex ualizationreport.files.wordpress.com/2013/12/thesex ualizationreport.pdf

14. Richens Y. *Investigation into fear of birth using a mixed methods design*. Unpublished PhD thesis. University of Manchester; 2016.

15. Fenwick J, Staff L, Gamble J, Creedy D, Bayes S. Why do women request caesarean section in a normal, healthy first pregnancy? *Midwifery*. 2010;26 (4):394–400.

16. Elharmeel S, Chaudhary Y, Tan S, Scheermeyer E, Hanafy A, van Driel M. Surgical repair of spontaneous perineal tears that occur during childbirth versus no intervention. *Cochrane Database of Systematic Reviews*. 2011; Issue 8; Art No. CD008534.

17. Menopause: Diagnosis and management. Nice.org.uk. 2015. Available from: www.nice.org.uk/guidance/ng23.

18. British Menopause Society. More than half of women feel negative about their experience of the menopause. London: British Menopause Society; 2017, 1–4. Available from: https://thebms.org.uk/2017/10/world-menopause-day-2/

how it develops during puberty, particularly if they are worried about how they look or feel. We hope it will reassure young people that vulvas come in a variety of shapes and sizes, and if they need advice and support, they can know where to go.

Labia Diversity Visuals: Books

The following books all feature varied collections of photographs of labia demonstrating the range of women's anatomy, with the aim of celebrating the differences and normal variation.

Femalia, Edited by Joanie Blank

Published 2011 by Last Gasp, USA

Joanie was an American sex educator, writer and editor, and supporter of the sex positive movement. She founded the Good Vibrations women-friendly adult store in San Francisco as well as her own publishing company called Down There Press. She was a great supporter of women and their freedom to express their sexuality. Notable honours include being granted an honorary Doctor of Arts by the Institute for Advanced Study of Human Sexuality in 2008 for her thirty years of work in sexuality.

Femalia is a book featuring thirty-two colour photographs of women's genitalia, edited by Joani. Femalia was a project she enjoyed and was proud to complete and make available to the world. It features photography by Michael Rosen, Jill Posener, Tee Corinne, Michael Perry and Joani herself.

I'll Show You Mine, Edited by Wrenna Robertson, Photographs by Katie Huisman

Published 2011 by Show Off Books, Canada

I'll Show You Mine features 120 photographs of 60 women in the same two positions. Each picture seeks to be as close to reality as possible, with life-size images in colour. Accompanying each woman's photos is text written by the woman, detailing her challenges and/or successes as pertains to her relationship with her genitals.

Women have long felt extraordinary pressure to conform to societal ideals of beauty. Digital alteration of photographs is rampant, and is now commonly used to alter the appearance of women's genitals. The labia minora (the inner lips of the vulva) are very frequently reduced, giving the vulva a "clamshell" or "Barbie Doll" appearance. As a result, viewing pornography may lead to a skewed understanding of the true diversity of the female anatomy.

This is particularly insidious as most women do not regularly have the opportunity to view other women's vulvas. This skewed understanding leads many women to feel that they are abnormal, leading to embarrassment, anxiety, and reduced genital self-image and overall self-confidence. The awareness of such procedures as labiaplasty can serve to further heighten women's belief that there is in fact a "normal", and that surgery is a suitable remedy for "abnormal" genitalia. Further, the practice of genital cosmetic surgery serves to promote a single genital morphology as ideal, in effect pathologizing natural diversity. Women must have the opportunity to view a range of diversity to gain an understanding that the societal ideal is an artificially created one, at the extreme end of the natural range of genital anatomy. However, there are very few resource tools available for women to gain a true appreciation of genital diversity. I created I'll Show You Mine to address this gap, to provide a resource that allows women and men (as well as boys and girls) to view a more representative sample of female genital diversity. The photographs in the book have not been altered in any way, and the accompanying narrative allows for a glimpse into each woman's complex relationship with her body.

– *Wrenna Robertson, editor of* I'll Show You Mine

Petals by Nick Karras

Published 2003 by Crystal River Publishing, USA

Petals is a collection of black-and-white photographs of labia by photographer Nick Karras. As well as the book, there is a poster of the images available which has been displayed in the offices of health practitioners.

When my mother found out that I was creating this book she asked, "why do you need to do this?". I got my first camera when I was 11 years old and discovered it was my way of relating to the outside world and showing others my perception of it. It was a natural fit for me to photograph everything around me.

In the late '90s the most incredible woman came into my life and became my lover. I soon discovered that hidden below all that beauty and power was a shame, almost disgust, for one part of her body, her vulva. With a lot of love, trust, and mutual respect, she allowed me to show her the beauty that I saw. She was so delighted and empowered by the journey we took in creating the image, she then showed it to a few of her girlfriends and the petals project was created. Over the last 10 years I have photographed over 250 women and it has been the most incredible experience. The

downloads/Labiaplasty%20%20final%20Position%20S
tatement.pdf

12. Rowen T, Gaither T, Awad M, Osterberg E, Shindel A, Breyer B. Pubic hair grooming prevalence and motivation among women in the United States. *JAMA Dermatol.* 2016;152(10):1106.

13. The sexualization report.Thesexualizationreport.files. wordpress.com. 2013. Available from: https://thesex ualizationreport.files.wordpress.com/2013/12/thesex ualizationreport.pdf

14. Richens Y. *Investigation into fear of birth using a mixed methods design.* Unpublished PhD thesis. University of Manchester; 2016.

15. Fenwick J, Staff L, Gamble J, Creedy D, Bayes S. Why do women request caesarean section in a normal, healthy first pregnancy? *Midwifery.* 2010;26 (4):394–400.

16. Elharmeel S, Chaudhary Y, Tan S, Scheermeyer E, Hanafy A, van Driel M. Surgical repair of spontaneous perineal tears that occur during childbirth versus no intervention. *Cochrane Database of Systematic Reviews.* 2011; Issue 8; Art No. CD008534.

17. Menopause: Diagnosis and management. Nice.org.uk. 2015. Available from: www.nice.org.uk/guidance/ng23.

18. British Menopause Society. More than half of women feel negative about their experience of the menopause. London: British Menopause Society; 2017, 1–4. Available from: https://thebms.org.uk/2017/10/world-menopause-day-2/

Appendix: Resources

Curated by Jennifer Beale

Introduction

This book has highlighted the need for appropriate and accurate information to support adolescent girls and women with concerns about their genital appearance as well as the health professionals involved in their management. While there is still a need for further development of resources, a variety of materials already exist which can be used in a clinical and educational context.

This section of the book lists labial diversity visuals under the following headings:

- Available on the internet as websites and blogs
- Published as books
- Sculpture
- Film

I have included a brief description of each resource. In addition I contacted all authors and offered them the opportunity to provide a brief description of their resource.

I have also included a section of supporting information for professionals:

- Professional Guidance

This list is not exhaustive and there may be other useful resources which have been overlooked or were still under development at the time this information was compiled. However, this does provide a useful starting board. All website details were up-to-date at the time of publication.

Labia Diversity Visuals
Websites and Blogs

In the modern age of the World Wide Web a wealth of information is just a click away. The following websites and blogs have been created by those interested in providing the public with access to labia diversity visuals in a non-sexual context. The websites contain content that is more than just photographs of labia, as explained in the following.

Keeping in mind the speed in which the online world evolves daily, at the time of curating this resource list the URLs linked below were up to date.

The Labia Library Website

www.labialibrary.org.au

Developed by Women's Health Victoria, a not-for-profit organization in Australia, the Labia Library website was developed in response to media reports about women seeking female genital cosmetic surgery. The website is visually appealing and easy to navigate, making it suitable for a broad audience. It contains information on 'everything you need to know about your labia' and a photo gallery of female genitalia taken from both "front and below" (standing and from between the legs). The photo gallery features forty colour photos of labia taken from the book *I'll Show You Mine* (see Books section) and provides an easy-to-access resource demonstrating labial diversity.

The website also has an 'Info and Advice' section for those wanting to seek advice from a medical practitioner about their labia, with links to other organisations with complementary advice on sex, relationships, and mental health.

The Labia Project: Body Positive Blog

www.labiaproject.com

Clare is based in Australia and has created The Labia Project: Body Positive blog. She posts comments, questions and photos of labia submitted by women all over the globe, and blogs about many topics related to the labia including female genital cosmetic surgery. Her blog contains a wide range of photos taken by adult women of their own genitalia. The words that accompany the photos reveal the everyday thoughts and questions from women in the present day.

There is a large amount of misinformation among women about what is 'normal' when it comes to the images are used in women's studies and empowerment workshops, sex education classes, and Ob/Gyn exam rooms, inspiring new and enlightening conversations. One of the models said to me "My mother once told me that much of the pain that women endure in life is centered in this most amazing of places, and yet it is often the last place we look for solutions. Fortunately, someone helped me to look in the right place by unfolding my petals".

— *Nick Karras, photographer and creator of* Petals

Heart of the Flower: The Book of Yonis by Andrew Barnes and Yvonne Lumsden

Published 2007 by Pangia Publishing Foundation, Australia

Heart of the Flower is a book of colour photographs of fifty women's vulvas combined with colourful imagery and floral photographs. The images draw on parallels between the vulva and flowers. In addition, alongside the photos, each woman writes about her relationship with her vulva.

I prefer to refer to our vaginas and vulvas as a 'yoni' – which can be loosely translated in Sanskrit as 'divine passage'. This book has a profoundly heartfelt reason for being and serves a number of noble purposes. Women of all ages, curious to learn more about their bodies in relation to other women's can do so in a healthy and empowering way. Likewise, men will also learn about the beauty and diversity of women's intimate anatomies.

Many women have not seen another woman's yoni, and wonder if their own looks 'normal' or whether it should be hidden and ignored. Or they may be one of an increasing number of women viewing pornography on screen or in magazines. Inevitably comparisons arise, and what most men and women don't realise is that many images of vulvas have been photoshopped to look a particular way.

There was a call to action from Consultant Clinical Psychologist Dr Liao and Consultant Gynaecologist Professor Creighton in the UK that in light of the increasing numbers of women seeking cosmetic genital surgery that women needed to see more positive and natural imagery of what other women's genitals looked like. Andrew and I answered the call and co-created Heart of the Flower – the book of yoni.

–*Yvonne Lumsden, Co-creator of*
Heart of the Flower: The Book of Yonis

Labia Diversity Visuals: Sculpture
The Great Wall of Vagina by Jamie McCartney

The Great Wall of Vagina features 400 plaster casts of female genitals by artist Jamie McCartney. The participants are from 18 to 76 years of age and show a wide range of anatomy, including a mother and daughter, twins, a woman during and after her first pregnancy, and post-vulval surgery.

In 2006 I was commissioned to make a large panel of plaster casts of genitals for a sex museum. The women who came to be cast for this sculpture would immediately examine the casts of the other women who had come before them and say things like, "Oh my God! I had no idea they looked so different" and "I wish mine looked like that one" or "I feel better about mine now". I knew men that worry unduly about their penises but I had no idea that genital anxiety amongst women was a thing.

As an artist it really piqued my interest that this casting process was having such a profound effect on my models. I realised this was the first time most of these women had had the opportunity to see what other women looked like down there. It is human nature to want to know where we fit in but for most men and women their only reference for other people's genitals was pornography, which has a rather narrow and distorted view of genital variety.

In my research I also discovered that cosmetic labia surgeries were the fastest growing cosmetic procedure in the UK. I was shocked. I didn't want to be a part of a society which was encouraging women to cut off parts of their genitals. That increasing numbers of women are deciding that they are 'defective' down there is terribly sad. I decided to set out to produce a sculpture that, via comparative castings, would demonstrate the huge variety of vulvar and labial shapes and sizes. The idea was that having seen it, nobody would have to worry about their 'bits' again. As an artist I saw this as a unique opportunity to make a powerful statement and a spectacular work of art, which would actually change people's lives.

— Jamie McCartney, artist and
creator of The Great Wall of Vagina

Documentary Films
The Centrefold Project by Ellie Land

The Centrefold Project is an award-winning animated documentary project exploring the increasing trend in women undergoing female genital cosmetic surgery. Funded by the Wellcome Trust, directed by filmmaker Ellie Land and partnered with clinicians from University College London Hospital, this project features two documentary films: *Centrefold* and *What the Experts Say.*

Centrefold is an animated documentary film presenting the personal accounts of three women who have had a female genital cosmetic surgery. The aim was to show a range of responses to labial surgery and a balance of views in order to promote informed thinking. A second film, *What the Experts Say,* provides commentary from Professor Sarah Creighton (gynaecologist) and Dr Lih-Mei Liao (psychologist) expanding on the information in the animated film from a medical and psychological viewpoint.

The films can be watched at http://thecentrefold project.virb.com

Petals: The Journey

A documentary film about the *Petals* project by Nick Karras (see earlier for details of the *Petals* book). *Petals: The Journey* is a film featuring interviews with sex educators, artists, cultural anthropologists, participants in the book, gynecologists, lesbian groups, and most importantly, the perspective of everyday people. It has been viewed in more than twenty-two countries by millions of people.

For more information on the documentary film, go to www.petalsthejourney.com.

Professional Guidance
Statements from Professional Bodies

- **British Society for Paediatric and Adolescent Gynaecology (BritsPAG)**

 October 2013 Position statement: " Labia reduction surgery (labiaplasty) on adolescents" October 2013

 Access the full paper at: www.rcog.org.uk/globalas sets/documents/news/britspag_labiaplastyposi tionstatement.pdf

- **Royal College of Obstetricians and Gynaecologists (RCOG) – Ethical Opinion Paper**

 October 2013 Ethical Considerations in relation to female genital cosmetic surgery

 Access the full paper at: www.rcog.org.uk/globalas sets/documents/guidelines/ethics-issues-and-resou rces/rcog-fgcs-ethical-opinion-paper.pdf

- **American College of Obstetricians and Gynaecologists – Committee Opinion**

 January 2017 Breast and labial surgery in adolescents

 Access the full statement at:

 www.acog.org/Resources-And-Publications/Com mittee-Opinions/Committee-on-Adolescent-Healt h-Care/Breast-and-Labial-Surgery-in-Adolescents

- **Society of Obstetricians and Gynaecologists Canada – Policy Statement**

 December 2013 Female Genital Cosmetic Surgery

 Access the full statement at:

 https://sogc.org/wp-content/uploads/2013/09/Dece mber2013-CPG300-ENG-Online_final.pdf

 Also published online in the *Journal of Obstetrics and Gynaecology Canada*. December 2013, Volume 35, Issue 12, pp. 1108–1112. www.jogc.com/article/ S1701-2163(15)30762-3/fulltext

- **Royal Australian and New Zealand College of Obstetricians and Gynaecologists – Statement**

 March 2015, "Vaginal 'rejuvenation', laser ablation for benign conditions and cosmetic vaginal procedures"

 Access the full statement at: www.ranzcog.edu.au/R ANZCOG_SITE/media/RANZCOG-MEDIA/Wom en%27s%20Health/Statement%20and%20guide lines/Clinical%20-%20Gynaecology/Vaginal-rejuve nation,-laser-and-cosmetic-procedures-(C-Gyn-24)- Amended-July-2016.pdf?ext=.pdf

Index